UNITAS:

HISPANIC AND BLACK CHILDREN IN A HEALING COMMUNITY

UNITAS:
HISPANIC AND BLACK CHILDREN IN A HEALING COMMUNITY

by
Anne Farber, Ph.D.,
Research Associate, Hispanic Research Center,
and Assistant Professor, Department of Sociology and Anthropology,
Fordham University,

and
Lloyd H. Rogler, Ph.D.,
Albert Schweitzer Professor of Humanities,
Fordham University.

Schenkman Publishing Company, Inc.,
Cambridge, Massachusetts

Schenkman Publishing Company, Inc.
3 Mount Auburn Place
Cambridge, Massachusetts 02138

ISBN 0-87073-505-5
ISBN 0-87076-506-3 (paper)

Printed in the United States of America

TABLE OF CONTENTS

PREFACE TO THE FIRST EDITION

Shortly after the establishment of the Hispanic Research Center in the fall of 1977, Dr. Edward Eismann -- founder and director of Unitas -- visited my office to request advice on research he felt compelled to undertake. He showed me some newspaper articles describing Unitas as a therapeutic outreach program serving Hispanic and black children in the South Bronx. He explained the concept of Unitas and what it attempted to do for the children. However, now his problem was that the funding agencies which had been financially supporting Unitas insisted upon evidence of Unitas' effect upon children. They wanted evaluation research which would demonstrate whether or not Unitas was attaining its goal of improving the mental health of the participating children. Their requests -- and strong insistence upon evaluation research -- responded to a rising pattern of concerns among public and private funding agencies regarding the need to document the impact of grant monies. Eismann's reaction to such pressures, in turn, was understandable. Following the prevailing methodological views of evaluation research, he had developed many scales purported to measure the personality dimensions of children. Now he wanted advice on the different time periods and different social situations in which to administer the scales in an effort to approximate a quasi-experimental research design. Such a design would yield inferences regarding the therapeutic impact of Unitas, which was the information sought by the funding agencies.

At Eismann's invitation, I visited Unitas one afternoon when an extended family circle meeting was being held. The symbolic families, composed of teenagers serving as surrogate parents, aunts and uncles, and the children, were assembled in circular fashion in a school gymnasium where Unitas meets during the school year. All together, one hundred and fifty-five youngsters, under Eismann's guidance, and the guidance of their surrogate parents, were discussing and analyzing problems, taking turns in expressing their views and in making observations of what was going on, many of them with their attention transfixed by the rich symbolisms of Unitas' rituals. There was a sense of discipline and of brotherly love and responsibility. Mutual help was emphasized as a means of healing the emotional hurts and injuries of childhood. Much of what I observed, however, I could not understand because of the subtle and intricate interactions. I found out that the extended family circle meeting in the school was held once a week during the school year, and four times a week in the summer in a street in the South Bronx cordoned off for this purpose. Such meetings were but one part of the Unitas program. Many other things were being done. Unitas, in brief, was a complicated institutional structure based upon philosophical, psychological, and sociological views of how interpersonal relations could be shaped in the interest of a child's healthy social life. To decipher it and understand it would take a special kind of research effort. Personality scales -- no matter how many or how often they were administered to the children -- would not yield an understanding of Unitas as an institutional structure with its own norms and values.

In my talks with Eismann I proposed the need to study Unitas as an institutional structure and that the fulfillment of such a need could complement the quasi-experimental designs used in the evaluation research. The understanding of changes over time in scale scores measuring dimensions of the children's personality, or differences in such scores from one situation to the next, would be enhanced if we understood Unitas as an intricate institutional structure impinging upon the children. I also proposed to Eismann that such a study could have considerable value in informing mental health workers about how one innovative, child-oriented outreach program operated in the South Bronx, an area which has come to symbolize the quintessence of urban decay in the United States. Perhaps mental health workers elsewhere in the country would then seek to replicate components of Unitas in economically disadvantaged urban neighborhoods. Eismann associated my proposal with humanistically oriented research, and agreed with the plan that the recently formed Hispanic Research Center undertake an ethnographic documentation of Unitas. The purpose would be to observe, describe, and analyze Unitas as a sociocultural system specifically designed to be of therapeutic help to children. I agreed to accept requests to explain to the representatives of the funding agencies how the study fit into evaluation research, and how such a study could make a solid contribution to our knowledge of therapeutic modalities.

My own interest in Unitas was based on several considerations and past experiences. Years before I had welcomed the rise of the community mental health movement and worked to develop community mental health centers in Puerto Rico. This attraction was based upon the sociological view that human interactions in society at large often contain elements of therapy or -- in the larger sense of the concept as used in Unitas -- of healing. Without doubting that society often and at times even relentlessly inflicts serious psychological injury upon the person, I believed, too, in the healing, restorative potential imbedded in human interactions. I recalled the pioneering research that the late Professor August B. Hollingshead and I had conducted in the slums and public housing developments in San Juan, Puerto Rico, on persons who suffered severe emotional problems and had no professional care. The research documented the therapeutic functions of spiritualist sessions in the contacts between the emotionally troubled person, on the one hand, and the medium and the other persons in the spiritualist session, on the other hand. Socially supportive therapy was also provided by concerned relatives and good friends. The capacity for therapy, I believed, was not the unique possession of a professional group, although distinctive types of training are associated with such groups. The capacity is in society at large, in the quality and form of human interactions imbedded in role relationships. To me, then, the community mental health movement represented along one dimension a nationwide effort to mobilize and organize much of what society already contained with the primary although not exclusive purpose of ameliorating the pervasive emotional distress of persons living in economically impoverished catchment areas. However, much of what I came to see evolving in community mental health centers in the United States mainland and in Puerto Rico itself did not represent efforts at such mobilization. Community mental health centers usually employed traditional therapeutic methods in the new catchment areas and seldom did I observe efforts made to change such methods -- or, for that matter, create new ones -- to better fit the sociocultural characteristics and service needs of the people in the new catchment areas. When the catchment area is composed of an economically disadvantaged migrant population from a different culture and speaking a different language -- such as the Hispanics living in the South Bronx -- the need to adapt service delivery becomes vitally necessary. It is not surprising, therefore, that whatever the specific reasons may have been, Eismann could not fulfill his abiding desire to help children within the organizational structure of a local community mental health center in the South Bronx. He was obliged to go to the streets of the South Bronx in order to reach out to the children and build a therapeutic structure to service their needs. In doing this he used old ideas, some of them tracing back to the vision of Maxwell Jones' therapeutic community which sees the potential for therapy in all human interactions. He imbedded these ideas in an innovative institutional structure. This attracted the attention of the newly formed Hispanic Research Center.

Unitas' focus upon children also coincided with the priority concerns of the Hispanic Research Center. The relevant research literature consistently indicates that social stress, as an external configuration of events imposing severe adaptational demands upon persons, is not randomly distributed in society. Persons in the lower levels of the socioeconomic structure are exposed to it in disproportionate amounts. So are migrants who enter host societies with a different language and culture. In fact, were one to deduce from the relevant research literature those conditions conducive to the experience of stress, a frightening similarity would be found between those conditions and the demographic profile and life experiences of New York City's Puerto Ricans. The stress model, in brief, fits the socially, culturally and economically marginated status of the city's Puerto Ricans. Moreover, longitudinally collected data indicate that in comparison to other groups the city's Puerto Ricans are experiencing a decreasing level of economic well-being in the midst of a society which emphasizes progress and upward mobility.

At the same time, the relevant literature also indicates that the connection between stress and the eruption of emotional problems in the person is *not* direct and immediate. The connection is mediated by the interaction of psychological, social, and cultural elements. Of paramount importance are those elements which enmesh the person in socially supportive interpersonal networks. The implicit hypothesis in all this is that persons who are strongly integrated into socially supportive networks -- the family, circles of friends, religious and other groups, the ritual coparent system of Hispanics *(compadrazgo)*, and perhaps a therapeutic community such as Unitas -- are better able to withstand the pressures of stress. In brief, the idea is that supportive networks mitigate the impact of stress.

To me, it was a matter of considerable interest that Eismann's creation of Unitas took as a point of departure the premise that the children drawn into Unitas came from families experiencing upheaval and disorganization. The families' potential for providing social support for the children, he believes, is minimal, and they could in fact represent a major source of stress for the children. Regardless of the truth of such premises, Unitas did represent a self-conscious effort to provide children with a set of supportive experiences to compensate for the dysfunctions attributed to their actual families. It was as if Eismann were taking hypotheses from the relevant literature as a prescription to plan his life's work: the creation and management of Unitas. Unitas was purposefully established as a tangible institutional derivative of beliefs and assumptions of far-reaching consequences. The Hispanic Research Center welcomed the many challenges of making systematic ethnographic sense out of such an innovative organization.

Perhaps it is somewhat ironic that the basic method used in studying Unitas -- participant observation -- contributed to the decision to conduct the research. One generally thinks of the research problem first and then decides upon the best and most efficient data collection procedures, and this perhaps is the way it usually ought to be. In our case our interest in a method, participant observation, and its importance in the program of evolving research of the recently formed Hispanic Research Center influenced the decision to study Unitas. As the director of the then neophyte center, I anticipated the development of many research projects in the future which would be based upon the analysis of secondary data, sample surveys, field experiments, controlled case studies, and so on. I was concerned that such studies, representing as they do, the prevailing and most powerful methodologies of the contemporary social sciences, would tend programmatically but inadvertently to push out studies based upon the essential act of directly observing the social field under study. In the very same way in which Eismann, not surprisingly, turned immediately toward the construction of personality scales in response to pressures from the funding agencies, the work of the center, I felt, would tend toward studies inevitably yielding quantifiable results. Important studies not yielding such results could be neglected. Generally, but not as a matter of methodological principle, participant observation does not yield quantifiable findings; and, as institutional structures, research centers orient themselves toward what they are best prepared to do which, at present, is the computer processing of data, not the interpretive examination of large masses of qualitative observational reports. I believe that the introduction of measurement and statistical models into the social sciences represents significant scientific progress. I believe equally strongly, however, that there will always be a major role to be played by the intrepid observer interested in making conceptual sense out of some comparatively small sociocultural system, without placing primary reliance upon data collection instruments independently developed and separate from the self. In participant observation the observer *is* the vehicle for registering observation. Thus, in the interest of incorporating into the center's work the diverse methodologies of the social and behavioral sciences, I was particularly interested in the prospect of an ethnographic study of Unitas.

The study was fortunate to have as an investigator Dr. Anne Farber who had recently joined Fordham University's Department of Sociology and Anthropology. A Columbia University trained anthropologist, she had conducted field research in the interior of Guatemala and was fluent in Spanish, an important asset because of the Hispanic children in Unitas. She not only had the requisite knowledge and skills to study Unitas but she was also a person gifted with the interpersonal sensitivity and competence the study demanded. Dr. Farber made the observations upon which the study is based and drafted the preliminary report. Throughout the study we had extensive and numerous collaborative discussions in making decisions and interpretations and in arriving at new formulations. We shared in the rewriting of the manuscript and in the honing of the final draft.

Chapter I of the monograph describes the organizational structure of Unitas including the temporal and spatial ordering of the program's activities and the composition of the Unitas professional staff, its teenage workers, and its participating children. Chapter II describes the Unitas concept of psychological healing and the two interpersonal methodologies Unitas uses -- and has innovatively adapted to its own needs -- to promote healing: the therapeutic community modality and psychotherapy. A discussion of the specific therapeutic systems and techniques developed by Unitas to treat its children is found in Chapter III. Chapter IV traces the beginnings of Unitas to its roots in the history of the community mental health movement and describes the personal development of Edward Eismann as the founder and director of the Unitas program. Chapter V provides a discussion of the justification for the creation of an elaborate symbolic family structure, clarifying the workings of Unitas, its hierarchical structure, and its impact on the lives of its teenage workers and children. Chapter VI briefly discusses the success of Unitas as a mental health program and the feasibility and desirability of replicating such a program.

This monograph is the sixth in a series published by the Hispanic Research Center to stimulate interest in Hispanic concerns. The first monograph reported on the health conditions of New York City's Puerto Ricans; the second presented a study of the outgroup marriage patterns of New York City's Hispanic populations; the third examined the Hispanic experience of the criminal justice system in the United States; the fourth appraised the mental health status and needs of Puerto Rican children in the New York City area; and the fifth examined the adaptation and adjustment of a large group of Cuban migrants living in West New York, New Jersey.

The Hispanic Research Center was established at Fordham University in 1977, under a grant from the National Institute of Mental Health, to work toward five major objectives: (1) to conduct interdisciplinary research on issues relevant to the mental health of the Hispanic population; (2) to increase and upgrade the number of Hispanic scholars experienced in doing research in the mental health-related disciplines; (3) to provide technical assistance to Hispanic behavioral scientists, professionals, and organizations interested in the mental health problems of Hispanic communities; (4) to develop links between individual Hispanic researchers and between these researchers and persons involved in the formulation and implementation of Hispanic relevant public policy; and (5) to disseminate information on the mental health of the Hispanic population.

We hope this monograph will be of general value to persons interested in the welfare of all children and of specific help to those persons who attend to the emotional needs of minority children.

Lloyd H. Rogler
Fordham University
January 1981

PREFACE TO THE SECOND EDITION

In keeping with one central objective of Fordham University's Hispanic Research Center (HRC), that of focusing its research to inform public policy and practice, the findings and recommendations in this report were widely disseminated. Almost without exception, the response to our research on Unitas was enthusiastic. The attention of readers of the monograph was caught by the innovativeness of the Unitas therapeutic community operating in the South Bronx; its work with emotionally distressed Hispanic and Black children living in deteriorated neighborhoods; its mobilization, recruitment, and training of teenagers from such neighborhoods to serve both as surrogate parents and as therapists to the children; the ingenious use of the concepts of fictive nuclear and extended families as the foundation of the program's social organization; the diverse ways in which the rituals enacted at Unitas' meetings, so deeply absorbing to the participating children, provide institutional meaning to the Unitas pattern of mutual help; the commitment to heal the psychological wounds resulting from a disadvantaged childhood; the cost-effectiveness of the Unitas program at a time of depleting budgets for inner-city programs; and, the vision of the founder and director of Unitas, Dr. Edward Eismann. Under his leadership, Unitas grew out of the grassroots of the South Bronx, to serve the emotional well-being of the neighborhood's children. All of this evoked the interest of those who through our research became familiar with Unitas.

This response, however, diverted attention from other issues of central concern to the Hispanic Research Center; issues centering upon the appropriate research methods to be used in such studies. From the preface to the first edition which follows, the reader will note the context of our decision to employ participant observation as the primary means for collecting data in the Unitas study, even though Dr. Eismann was being pressured by the organizations funding Unitas to conduct psychological evaluations of the impact of the program upon the participating children. We believed that participant observation should be one of the data collection methods forming part of the research of the recently established HRC. Also, we looked upon this technique, tactically, as the first step in a comprehensive, well-rounded evaluation of the Unitas experience. Our reasons were straightforward: although not a large-scale bureaucracy, Unitas is an institutional structure with diverse therapeutic modalities and patterns of participation. In the absence of an ethnographic study based upon participant observation, quasi-experimental research framed exclusively to identify psychological change and continuity in the Unitas children would yield findings incapable of interpretation in the context of Unitas. Such studies, in general, inevitably yield mixed findings: some of the attributes of the participants change in the desired direction, others do not. To reasonably interpret such findings, indeed, even to raise sensible questions about them, much has to be known about the participants themselves and about the institution which impinges differentially upon them. Persons learning of our research, however, riveted their attention upon Unitas and not upon our own methodological preoccupations. Perhaps this was indicative of the study's success: we had rendered such a comprehensive account of the program as to make issues of methodology of trivial importance in the audience's mind. As tempting as this self-congratulatory explanation might be to the authors, it must quickly give way to one which is far more plausible: the audiences focused exclusively upon the substance of Unitas and not upon the procedures for its study because Unitas is of itself a topic of compelling interest.

But the audiences were not uncritical. Questions were raised about Unitas. Perhaps it would be instructive to discuss briefly some of these questions, since they may possibly foreshadow issues which will arise in the reader's mind as he or she proceeds through this account.

Questions were raised about the apparent religious, cult-like quality of Unitas, and in one case, associations were drawn with movements such as that of Sun Myung Moon and the now extinguished Jonestown establishment in Guyana, South America. The reader will note, in fact, that much of what occurs in Unitas has a kind of religious flavor -- there is incessant attention given to the ethical responsibility of helping others (although this ethic, of course, is not exclusively religious) and to the enactment of rituals, some of which derive from Judeo-Christian traditions. Also, the demeanor of the Unitas founder and director, Dr. Edward Eismann, imparts an aura of benevolent reverence. Unitas, however, differs fundamentally from cult-like movements. As is true of all social systems, Unitas' activities create boundaries around itself. Nonetheless, while retaining its identity as an institutional structure, Unitas seeks to enmesh itself into the surrounding community in myriad ways by working with neighborhood-based mothers' groups and local schools, by the actions of its participants returning to their homes every day, and through the outward reaching activities of its therapeutically trained cadre of teenagers. Cult-like movements develop mechanisms to perpetuate their differentiation and isolation from the external world in order to monopolize internally the power of sanctions in the enforcement of organizational discipline. Unitas seeks no such isolation, nor does it seek such centralized control over its participants.

Unitas differs from cults, too, in its basic orientation toward performance in the outside world. It views itself as preparatory, as a school which imparts skills, values, and attitudes which will be helpful elsewhere in the future lives of the children and teenagers.

Questions were also raised about the organization's therapeutic theories. In this regard, it is perhaps more than a matter of passing interest that even though Eismann uses the word "healing" in response to the need to mend the psychological wounds of children of the ghetto, he self-consciously avoids reference to "sick behavior" or to "emotionally sick" children. This is true even though one-third to one-half of the children participating in Unitas have been so labelled in the outside world. No references to schizophrenia, cyclothymic personalities, depressive psychotics, psychopathic disorders will be found in this report, nor, for that matter, will there even be allusions to the nomenclature of psychiatric discourse. Such concepts are anathema to the therapeutic premises of Unitas, implying as they do a model of mental illness which entrenches sickness in the character of the person. Though recognition is given to acting-out, bizarre, and withdrawn behaviors in Unitas, such behaviors are viewed as variants of being "misguided." The very word itself -- misguided -- implies that incorrect or wrong guidance has been given to the children. Unitas' task, then, is to redirect the child, to guide him or her correctly. This is to be done by teaching skills, values, and attitudes conducive to participation in the broader segements of American life.

Other questions raised the possibility of apparently damaging contradicitons in what Unitas strives to impart to the children in relation to their lives in the South Bronx. Quick recourse to physical violence or to physical aggression toward other persons generally or toward persons whose conduct is seen as provoking, is one important target of Unitas' effort to redirect the misguided child. An outburst of violence is quickly seized upon as an opportunity to teach and to learn the underlying interpersonal processes which gave rise to it. Under the tutelage of the more experienced participants, the process is analyzed to uncover the precipitants of the outburst, to lay bare the latent meanings imbedded in the situation, and to understand empathically the reciprocal feelings of the participants or opponents. The process is framed to show that insightful understanding expressed through the medium of talk can assuage exacerbated feelings, diminish tension, and avert violence. To some of the questioners, it appeared that all of this could render the properly instructed Unitas child defenseless in neighborhoods where violence is seemingly institutionalized. The point of the question is too complex to enable a complete and satisfactory answer, assuming as it does much about the habitual responses acquired by the children as a result of participating in Unitas and much, too, about the children in relation to the South Bronx neighborhood environment. But one answer provided by a representative from Unitas may be of interest to the reader: "... the children of Unitas already know how to fight. They need no further instruction in fighting." Unitas imparts to them a peaceful alternative to the solution of tension-provoking situations.

Another important question concerns the capability of Unitas teenagers to serve as paraprofessional therapists in their relationship to the younger children. This question calls attention to the central role teenagers played in the history of Unitas and continue to play. The rise of Unitas as an organizational structure began when Dr. Eismann formed strong bonds of friendship with a small group of teenagers, reinforcing their personal friendships with each other and with himself. This core group recruited other teenagers in the neighborhood to join them in working together with children. At the same time, the capacity of the teenagers to move into the lives of children was directly related to the caring they themselves received from Dr. Eismann and the emerging social organization of Unitas. As he dealt with them, so they dealt with others. Thus, Unitas was not formed as a bureaucratic response to the perceived emotional needs of children, nor were there a series of official guidelines laid down as in the formation of bureaucratic organizations. Rather, Unitas was the result of a grassroot working alliance between the teenagers themselves and between them and Dr. Eismann. To this day, the issue of Unitas' replicability rests upon the social mobilization of neighborhood teenagers into a therapeutically trained cadre of symbolic parents dedicated to the welfare of children in their neighborhoods.

Correlatively, the issue of the program's effectiveness rests upon the therapeutic capabilities of the teenagers and is premised upon the assumption that teenagers can be selected and trained to have such capabilities. The importance of this issue did not escape the attention of the researchers: the report is replete with descriptive accounts of the efforts made to select and train the teenagers and, beyond this, there is the likely operation of broadly selective processes which bring into Unitas teenagers disposed toward the performance of paraprofessional therapeutic roles. (Parenthetically, the Hispanic Research Center will soon publish a manual for the replication of the Unitas program, written by Dr. Edward Eismann, which will devote considerable attention to the training of teenagers). Even though there is a growing research literature on the effectiveness of paraprofessionals, the logically most satisfactory answer to this question cannot be provided at present in the absence of research testing for how children change, if at all, as a result of the Unitas experience. The reader will note in the preface to the first edition which follows that it was the need for such a study which first brough Unitas to our attention. The process of inquiry begins where another such process ends.

Lloyd H. Rogler
Director, Hispanic Research Center
Fordham University
April 1982

ACKNOWLEDGEMENTS

The research for this monograph was supported by the Hispanic Research Center of Fordham University. We wish to thank Dr. Edward Eismann and Ms. Lynn Stekas for the generous giving of their time and expertise which contributed to the accuracy of the data in this report and to many of its insights. They maintained their enthusiasm and support throughout the research and writing, and provided important introductions to children and teenagers, professionals and community leaders. Our special gratitude and admiration go to the teenagers of Unitas, particularly to Severo Escalera, for acting as a guide to the Unitas experience and its setting; James Arana, for welcoming us into his Unitas family; and Jose Luis Vargas, for his extra effort in assisting in the collection of data. The entire staff of Unitas, especially Wilson Martinez del Rio, provided invaluable information and assistance. Our warmest thanks go to the children of Unitas who allowed us to participate in their games, visit them in their homes, and welcomed us as part of the Unitas family.

Nannette Giunta gathered much of the data on the psychological aspects of Unitas and contributed significantly to the second and third chapters of this monograph. Lori Repetti provided all-around assistance in coordinating and organizing different phases of the project. Dr. Lilliam Barrios Paoli did helpful preliminary work on the project.

We are grateful to the hardworking staff of the Hispanic Research center who made the project run smoothly with their expert administrative, secretarial, and typing skills: Elizabeth Ospina, Mercedes River, Elizabeth Collado, and Magdalena Porata. Stasia Madrigal edited and nursed the manuscript from its first version to the final draft. We wish also to thank Kyonghee Min, Michael Vaccaro, and Kevin Colleran for their assistance with the statistical analysis. Edna Schroder and Elizabeth Collado provided invaluable assistance in preparing the preface to the second edition.

Discussions with colleagues helped us to formulate the direction and methods of this study. We thank Douglas Gurak, Rosemary Santana Cooney, Sheila Klatzky, and Charles Melville for their ideas and suggestions. Special thanks go to Richard Kaiser for his support and encouragement throughout the research and writing of this monograph.

Hispanic Research Center — *Anne Farber*
Fordham University
January 1981 — *Lloyd H. Rogler*

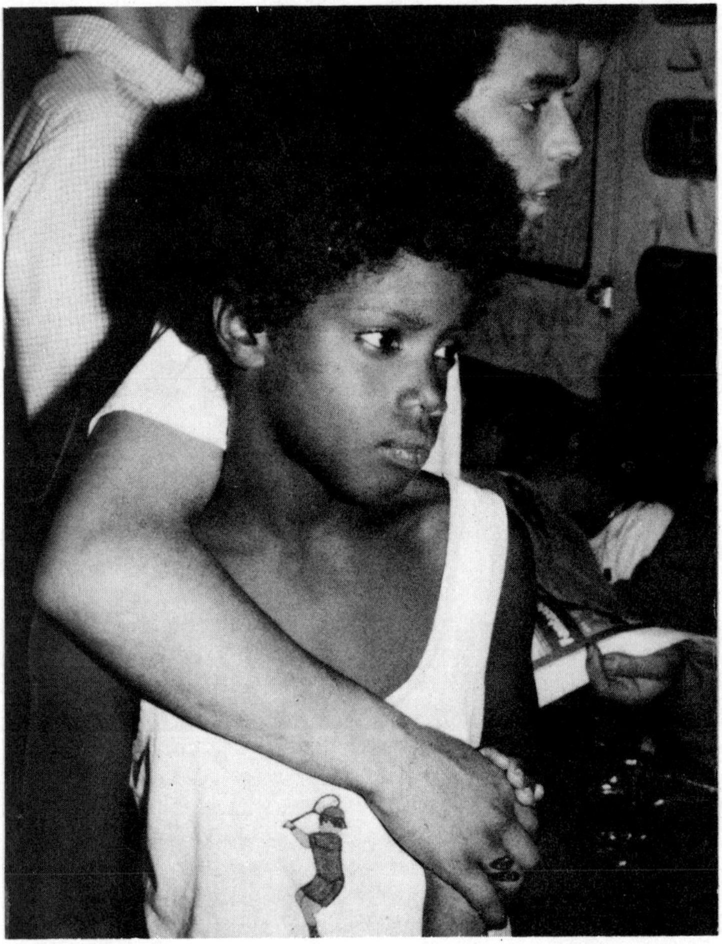

PLATE 1. "How good it is and how noble for brothers to live together in Unity." *Psalm 133*.

Dedicated to the teenagers of Unitas
who care for the children
on the streets of the South Bronx

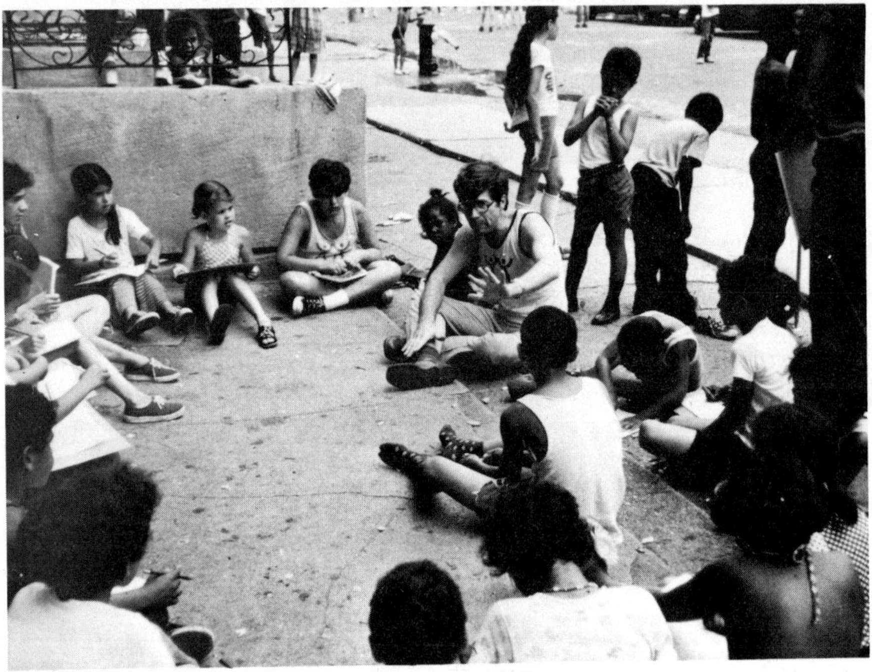

PLATE 2. Edward Eismann conducting an art group on Fox Street: establishing the parameters of boundary and order.

I

UNITAS STRUCTURE

Unitas is a mental health organization serving a predominantly Hispanic population of children in the Longwood/Hunts Point section of the South Bronx, an area which has become a nationwide symbol of economic and social decay. Unitas serves children and their families in an area where one out of three residents is on welfare and where the unemployment rate is from 20 to 30 percent. The area has the largest number of families headed by women and the largest child population in the Bronx.[1]

Unlike many community-based organizations, Unitas does not wait for troubled youth to knock at its door or to be remanded there for treatment of their mental ills. Each September, Unitas teenage workers and staff visit the teachers at the local elementary schools. The teacher, in conjunction with a Unitas worker, completes a Behavior Rating Checklist, indicating which children are troubled. The parents of these children are then contacted by staff members and, in some cases, by the teachers themselves. Referrals are also made by community helpers in churches, nearby schools, and local service agencies. Teenagers and children make up another source of referrals. Children who come to Unitas usually bring their siblings, other relatives, and their friends. Youth workers and staff also go out on the streets, talking with the people of the area with the aim of introducing children, teens, and parents to Unitas.

The Unitas program operates in two cycles corresponding to the school calendar. The bulk of its work takes place during the summer months when it can command the full attention of its school-age participants. In July and August, Monday through Friday, Unitas serves between 150 and 200 children aged 4 to 16, providing recreation in arts, crafts, and sports. These activities are

[1] *Research Bulletin*, Hispanic Research Center, Fordham University, Bronx, New York: April 1979.

only vehicles, however, for the more important work of Unitas, namely, therapeutic guidance and intervention. The stated goals of Unitas are far-reaching:

> ...to prevent, combat, and remediate family disintegration and other emotional and social problems of hard-to-reach youth and families.[2]

Of the approximately 200 children participating in Unitas, between one-third and one-half have been referred as problem children. Unitas uses three basic diagnostic procedures to distinguish troubled children from normal children: (1) withdrawn (quiet, immature, shy); (2) acting out (truant, fighting, disruptive, violent); and (3) atypical (bizarre, borderline, multiproblemed). The children referred to Unitas are treated as emotionally deprived, having received insufficient caring attention or suffered outright neglect or abuse, both psychological and physical. They are wanting a stable family structure, consistent discipline, and living routines such as regular meals, sleeping quarters, and supervision. As a result, they have low self-esteem; are distrustful of others; use inappropriate, often self-destructive or anti-social means of getting attention; have never learned to identify and accept their feelings or to control their impulses; and feel helpless and unloved. These children, in effect, do not have a family in the psychological sense. Unitas seeks to provide them, if not with a psychological family, then with therapeutic interventions aimed at re-parenting them and re-educating them emotionally.

To achieve this, Unitas has developed a "social-psychological intervention" which attempts

> ...to create a therapeutic climate in the child's natural milieu where order, nurturance, and discipline are developed and maintained for them.

Unitas sees the family unit as the basic and most important natural institution that can satisfy a child's need for nurturance, discipline, and belonging. However, traditional family therapy intervention is often not possible because "actual families may be so disrupted and disorganized that they are not accessible to change through family treatment." Unitas, therefore, has created a system of symbolic families composed of up to fifteen boys and girls, usually living on the same street, but not necessarily from the same family. Each symbolic family is headed by one or two older neighborhood teenagers who play the roles of symbolic mothers and

[2] This quotation and all others in this monograph, unless otherwise identified, come from the verbal communications, taped conversations, and the writings of Dr. Edward Eismann, founder and director of Unitas.

fathers. Supervised mainly by one another and by Dr. Edward Eismann, these older teenagers receive intensive training in psychological theory and clinical skills and become the primary caretakers, counselors and, indeed, therapists of the younger children. According to Eismann:

> The function of the surrogate parents *vis-a-vis* their symbolic children is to provide a corrective experience to them as well as non-punitive discipline, when needed, to offset the negative impact of the actual treatment they get at home which is not readily changeable.

Within this context, the primary role of the therapist is not to help the troubled children directly, but to create a climate so that the healthy children learn to have an influence on others. The older children are encouraged by their symbolic parents to nurture, discipline, and care for their younger symbolic siblings, thus creating a network of supervised, therapeutically oriented interaction. Within this system, Dr. Eismann plays the role of symbolic grandparent.

Once each week during the school year and four times each week during the summer months an extended family circle is held in a local school gym. These meetings are highly structured and ritualized; all children sit with their symbolic families which include symbolic parents, aunts, uncles, and children. Dr. Eismann leads discussions of a topic of his choosing such as friendship, or one raised by a family member, usually stemming from a specific problem or comment. Each extended family circle meeting is followed by play time in which children participate in activities such as baseball, jumprope, blocks, board games, volleyball, gymnastics, reading, or art. A regular staff member or a teen "parent" supervises each activity.

Responding to the existing institutional constraints on the children of the community, Unitas operates in two phases: a Summer program and a Fall-Winter-Spring program. These phases overlap in content, organization, and personnel, but are treated distinctly by all involved.

A. *The Summer Program*

The Summer Program begins in early July and ends in August. Registration begins in the last weeks of June and is an easy procedure. A parent fills out a simple form found at the bottom of a mimeographed flyer briefly describing the summer activities, giving the child's name and address, and returns this with one dollar to Unitas. There are no other fees for participation. Parents may also request more information, in which case they are contacted by a staff member. Unitas staff and teenagers are in charge of distributing flyers to classes at the two local elementary schools. There is no cut-off date for registration and, indeed, registration is not a requirement for participation. Most children come into the program by the time it begins functioning on its summer schedule, but they may also enter after the program begins.

Recruitment of teenagers to work during the summer as symbolic parents proceeds in a different way. All but eight of the more than thirty teenage and young adult workers in Unitas during the summer have been involved in the program previously. The new teenage workers are assigned before the start of the summer program by the New York City Youth Employment Program, which pays their weekly salaries. All other full-time staff members are paid by Unitas and do not change their status from one phase of the program to the other.

The day before the summer program officially begins, teen workers, regardless of their previous experience in Unitas, come to an all-day orientation meeting in St. Athanasius school where chairs have been arranged in a large circle around a classroom. Eismann starts the meeting by asking whether anyone knows why they are there. "To work," replies one boy. Eismann responds, "To work, that's the name of the game," and then introduces himself briefly. "I'm not the kind of doctor who gives injections. I help kids with their worries," he explains.

Eismann initiates activities that serve to ease the tension of the first day's lack of familiarity. He asks how many people know at least one person in the room, or two persons, no people, and so on. Next, he asks everyone to look at the floor and, one by one, estimate the number of people in the room. Then the teens count each other off. The remainder of the day is spent in going over the rules of the Youth Employment Program and of Unitas, the daily routine for the summer, becoming familiar with the other workers, and learning the style of the program. Rather than talk about the Unitas program at length or about the handling of difficult situations with children and coworkers, Eismann has the teens focus on their immediate interactions with one another. Some of the teens are noticeably bored by the focus on introspection, constant reiteration of what has just been said, and the need to help one another verbally. Eismann makes clear to the group that they are being tested to see who will be a good worker and who will not:

> We want to know who can speak up and command leadership. On the street we have children who need

> you. Because of the nature of the work you may feel uncomfortable about it if you're not used to it. We need to know how you'll perform. Help each other.

The teenagers are, indeed, being tested from the first day, and not all will pass. Eismann has discovered through the years that untrained, unresponsive teenagers can be more trouble to have around than not. In addition, the newly assigned teenagers will most likely not be in Unitas after the summer, making an investment of training and time in them even less desirable. If a teenager is perceived as unresponsive and non-interactive, and if this same teenager does not live in the immediate Unitas neighborhood or does not have previous involvement in the program, then he or she may well be dismissed.

By the end of the first day, all the teens have had the chance to talk with one another and the message has been delivered that

> ...in a group, any problem that any one person has affects the whole group. Like in a family. Since it affects everybody, everybody has a say in resolving the problem.

The themes of human interrelatedness and communication have been stressed repeatedly and consistently. The next few days will tell whether these messages of Unitas have been received and whether they will be heeded.

Orientation continues the next morning with the introduction of regular staff therapists who briefly describe the work they do. By noon, when they break for lunch and begin their work with the children, each teen has been assigned an activity for the afternoon and the remainder of the summer. For each activity there is at least one "old-timer" who can teach the newcomers the Unitas way.

The weekly summer calendar at Unitas combines day camp and therapy, the two usually taking place simultaneously. On Mondays, Wednesdays, and Fridays at 10 a.m. from 50 to 100 children usually congregate on a neighborhood street to leave for the Central Park swimming pool. Older teen workers lead the group to the subway station and supervise the morning's swimming activities. The children are back at St. Athanasius for lunch by 12:30 or 1 p.m. Lunch, provided free of charge by the Public School Lunch Program, is set up by the lunch crew composed of old-timer male teenagers picked by Eismann to do this job. These teenagers, supervised only minimally in their tasks, distribute lunches to the children and their symbolic parents as they file through the doors of the school gym. Upon getting a lunch, each person sits with his or her symbolic family in a large circle. Eismann emphasizes lunchtime as an important part of the teenager's work time with the children; the offering and sharing of food with others is seen as creating or reinforcing human intimacy. By 1:30 or 2 p.m. lunch and cleanup are over and a brief rest period begins. The children leave for home or for the streets, often with an extra piece of fruit or even a whole lunch to take to a sister or brother. Like the teenagers, they are free until the start of the afternoon program at 2:30.

Tuesdays and Thursdays are reserved for training the teenage workers in therapeutic philosophy and techniques. There are no formal activities for the children, although it is during these times that the full-time staff therapists make home visits to clients in the area. The training sessions begin at 10 a.m. and go on until noon, usually with a 10 to 15 minute break when fruit drinks and doughnuts are often provided. Eismann runs the training and usually devotes an entire morning to one theme, such as anger or the handling of fights between children. Eismann encourages the teens to draw on their own experiences with the children, with each other, and within their families in probing their feelings. The older, experienced teens are particularly helpful in these sessions since they usually sense what Eismann is aiming for and they work to move the group in the desired direction. An example of a typical interaction taken from a training session follows.

By 10 a.m. on a hot August day, the teens have gathered upstairs in the school. Doughnuts and Hawaiian Punch have been set out for them. After some preliminary business Eismann opens the floor to the workers saying:

> Now I'd like you to express the thoughts or feelings you have about your work and relationships together, your work with the children, assignments on the street. This is a time to talk together and share your points of view.

The discussion is initiated by Ricardo,[3] a newcomer to Unitas. Ricardo complains that when they play volleyball on the street, people on bikes and in trucks and cars pass by and break the volleyball net. Several teenagers suggest ways to handle this matter, e.g., assign teenagers to the end of the street to turn away vehicles or park a car across the end of the street. One teen recommends that they get the drivers to back down the street. This leads to the topic of communication and Juan, a teen "elder," focuses on the form of delivery of this or any message. Now Eismann breaks into the discussion.

[3] With the exception of the names of Edward Eismann and Lynn Stekas, Unitas administrator, all names of children and staff in this monograph have been changed to ensure confidentiality.

Eismann: It's all in the way you say things. We could say, "Call the police, and have them ticket every car. It's illegal for them to be there. Let the air out of their tires." It's really a matter of how you say things. How do you think the boys on the bike felt?

Jesus (a newcomer): Mischievous.

Raul (a young teen with experience in Unitas): Having fun, having a good time.

Eismann: What Juan said goes a little further than what the other brothers see. I think he's right. He's saying more than what he sees. Do you see the difference?

Raul: Try to empathize. Put yourself in the person's place.

Eismann goes around the room asking teenagers if they see how this is the same as what they have been doing as a group in Unitas. He calls on Susan, a quiet newcomer to Unitas, to repeat what Raul has just said. Unable to do this correctly, Susan, encouraged by Eismann and her coworkers, asks Raul to repeat what he has said. Eismann again requests a restatement of Raul's observation, this time from others. The theme of empathy is gradually developed, nurtured by Eismann's zeroing in on those comments which are most relevant.

After some observations by teens about their experiences with children, Janet relates Raul's remark to a discussion the group had had a week earlier in a training session.

Eismann (to Raul): How did you feel about Janet's statement?

Raul: That was it!

Eismann: She really understood you?

Raul: Yeah.

Eismann: How did that make you feel?

Raul: Like it was really cleared up.

Eismann (to everyone): What does this have to do with the boys on the bikes?

Mary (a newcomer): Ask the kids on the bikes what they might be feeling.

Eismann: The boys looked like they were having fun. What could you say to them?

Juan: You could say, "You look like you're having fun." Keep it short.

Eismann: You're not asking questions or telling them what to do. You're not punishing or threatening. You're helping to bring about cooperation. Do you see the point, Mary? You were almost there but we had to go over one more hurdle.

At this point Eismann calls for a break and suggests that they all move downstairs to the gym to escape the heat. The discussion resumes with Eismann asking how each teen would feel if he or she were the motorist on the block.

Eismann: Let's say you're the motorist on the block. You like the Unitas program, but you have to get your car out. How would you feel?

Tom (an experienced teen and Eismann's adopted son): I'd want to get out.

Eismann (to the others): Can you help Tom out?

Janet: I could ask him to move back.

Eismann: Sounds like what Tom said.

Frank (an experienced teen): You could say, "I understand how you feel."

Janet: "I know it's a hot day and I know that you don't want to move your car but..."

Eismann interrupts Janet abruptly, "Stop! You don't have to go further." Then, turning to the other teens, asks, "Why did I say that?"

Mary: You want her just to say what the feelings are.

Eismann: That's the most important part -- to understand. Now we need another motorist. We need a woman motorist.

Carlos, an old-timer in Unitas, reluctantly volunteers and is selected by Eismann to role-play a motorist, although there was a specific request for a female. Barbara, a newcomer, is asked by Eismann to take the role of the Unitas worker. Before beginning, Barbara and Carlos change roles and places in the group circle. Barbara temporarily plays the motorist. Eismann then describes a scene in which the motorist needs to use his car to go to work. The day is hot and humid and there are kids all over the car. Eismann then turns to Barbara (as motorist) and asks, "How are you feeling?"

Barbara: Miserable!

Eismann: Beautiful word.

Barbara and Carlos change places again. Barbara, now playing a Unitas worker, says to Carlos, "I know you feel miserable."

Eismann (to the group): These are the ways you might say it: "Wow, you must feel miserable." "I wouldn't be surprised if you really feel miserable." "If I were in your shoes, I'd really feel miserable." Do you see how the same feelings can be communicated in different ways? Using the word miserable, how else might you say it to the motorist?

Raul: Miserable day, isn't it?

Tom: What a miserable way to start out!

Eismann (to Tom): Say it to the motorist.

Tom (to Carlos): What a miserable way to start out!

Role-playing continues with different teenagers acting as bicyclist and worker. The teenagers, now understanding the types of responses most acceptable to Eismann, need little coaxing to play their roles well. Several teens begin to embellish the dialogue with wit and street language. The teens are relaxed and clearly enjoying themselves, laughing and applauding one another. As the excitement diminishes, Eismann summarizes and expands on what has just happened.

> The answer is in how you talk to people, that you know what it is to be in their shoes. The person may be depressed. Is there anyone who hasn't been there or hoped that something exciting would happen and was then disappointed? At those times what you need is someone to do for you what you have to do for another person now. This is the most human language to understand, one you learned as children but which you learned not to feel. We've been taught not to. We have to get back to the feeling of childhood, to use that with each other and with the children.

Finally, Eismann returns to Ricardo's original problem with the driver, bicyclists, and the volleyball net. He asks who in the group would be available to help Ricardo should this problem arise again. Ten people, about one-third of the teens present, raise their hands to volunteer. Ricardo chooses one teenager to whom he says he will turn for assistance. Eismann then tells the teens that he will intervene on the street when the workers appear to be having special problems with the children.

> It's one thing to talk about it and understand and another to put it into practice. This is called therapeutic communication.

During the remaining twenty minutes, several topics of a business nature are raised and handled. An important in-house problem having to do with the length of the work day is introduced but there is obvious reluctance on Eismann's part to deal with it then and there. In spite of Eismann's attempt to put off the discussion, Lynn Stekas, the Unitas administrator, insists that the problem be resolved immediately. Few feelings, however, are explored in the resolution process since it is getting late and all are anxious to leave for lunch.

Morning training sessions end a little after noon. Lunch for the children and teenagers follows, as it does on the other days when the group returns from the swimming pool. However, on training days, the teens have more free time between the end of lunch and the start of the afternoon program at 2:30. The teenagers' pay will be docked if they do not return in the afternoon, though it is only among a handful of the newly assigned teens that such a constraint is relevant. Most of the teens are pleased to participate in the program and devote extra hours on a voluntary basis to Unitas which speaks to the strength of the bonding engendered by the program. The children, too, have good attendance records for the summer program.

A little before 2:30 children begin to congregate on Fox Street, which has been closed to traffic for the Unitas afternoon program. As bats, balls, exercise mats, and arts and crafts materials appear, the children gradually settle into activities in the street, on stoops, and shaded corners. Eismann is rarely present for the start of the afternoon program; the teenagers take responsibility for planning activities and bringing out the necessary materials from St. Athanasius and the basement of a tenement which serves as their storage area on the street.

Teen workers have no say about the activities to which they are assigned, but may exchange activities with other teens. At the start of the summer, Eismann assigns one or more teens to one of thirteen activity areas. The division of assignments runs along traditional sex-role lines. Males handle basketball, wiffleball, plaster casting, painting, woodwork, dodgeball, and kickball. Females manage block building, lincoln logs, tinker toys, board games such as Monopoly and checkers, drawing with pencils and crayons, T-shirt and water cup table (shirts and plastic cups are silkscreened with the Unitas logo and sold for one dollar each), and jump rope. Three activities -- crafts, *decoupage* (a combination of woodworking and painting), and mats -- are managed by both males and females. The mat work, described by Eismann as one of the most important activities on the street, has generally been organized and run by more experienced male teens. It tends to attract more boys than girls. This year, while males still predominate in this activity in both staff and children, two female workers have been assigned to mats. Well aware of the difficulties in getting girls involved in mat work, Eismann explains to the teens:

> On mats particularly I want girls. Girls stay away from mats unless there's a woman. They stay away from gymnastics. Encourage them to have courage. Especially the girls. They're put down too much.

There are no equally explicit attempts to alter sex roles in other areas. Indeed, as indicated in the listing of the activities and their staff composition, Unitas, in its assignment of workers, has encouraged the separation of males and females and the continuation of traditional sex-role-oriented activites.

In spite of a seemingly rigid structure, Unitas gives ample opportunity to children and teens to structure their own time. Children are free to choose any of the organized activities or to play on their own by themselves or with friends. Teens do not have to attend to their activity areas exclusively. If they must leave their activity, especially to be with a child who needs their assistance, they may do so as long as their coworkers know where they have gone and agree to their leaving. Beyond signing in and out each day there are virtually no outside checks on the teens. They are expected and encouraged to be responsible to and for one another. If a teen shirks his or her duty, it is assumed that coworkers will deal appropriately with the problem.

Play activities continue until about 4:30 p.m. when cleanup begins. Eismann has been on the street for well over an hour by now, going from activity to activity, talking with the children, the teens, and the adults on the street. By 5 p.m. all materials are put away and children and workers move to their places on the street getting ready for the afternoon extended family circle.

By 5:10, if there is still commotion, Eismann speaks up, "I am waiting for the family to unite the people," or "I'll know by your silence when you are ready," or words to that effect. When the children and teens quiet themselves down, the afternoon extended family circle begins. This is a time for the children to speak their minds. Typically, the children tell briefly about something of interest happening at home, e.g., a visit by a relative from Puerto Rico, a misunderstanding between the speaker and another child, a complaint about Unitas, the loss of an item, or a query about a person absent from the group. Eismann deals with each comment or question. Often, the group spends considerable time helping the child to communicate his or her idea, e.g., to get Jimmy to speak loudly and clearly to Henry rather than direct his comment to Eismann. The main role of the other symbolic family members in this case might well be to help Jimmy to communicate effectively rather than to solve whatever problem he presents.

Generally, Eismann adjourns the meeting by 5:45. Children, some with crafts in hand from their afternoon's work, scatter quickly, as do teen workers who are anxious to end the work day. A number of teens, especially the old-timers, return to St. Athanasius to socialize for an hour or so with their friends after signing out for the day.

In the second half of the summer program, the full-time staff (including several of the older, experienced teens, but not the other teen workers) meet for one and a half hours to discuss scheduling problems, organization of the program, worker relations, and other business matters. This time is also used by the workers to bring complaints to Eismann on behalf of their more reticent, younger coworkers. The older teen workers often act as mediators between both the younger teens and the children and the administration, mainly Eismann.

The Unitas summer program is officially over at the end of August. It is followed by a period of several weeks in which there is no organized large group activity for the children. Individual and family therapy continues as the Unitas staff prepare for the winter program. Since workers and children are between programs and structures, as well as seasons, this is a time of flux and confusion. Not wanting to lose the momentum of the summer, Unitas struggles to keep its presence felt on the streets and in the minds of the children and teens. To assure continuity, Eismann directs the staff to "go to the street and hang around...have contacts with teens. Unitas is not just when the program is in action but whenever people are together." Staff members suggest simple activities -- tossing a football or playing a game of cards -- that they may take out to the street to maintain the continuity that Eismann wants.

From mid-September to the end of October, or whenever the cold weather drives people inside, Unitas holds extended family circle meetings, complete with preceding play activities, on the street. Several weeks after school begins, Unitas sends out envoys to describe the program to teachers and guidance counselors and to ask for referrals of problem children. The children referred in this way will be seen individually by one of the mental health workers, in their school, within the context of their real family, or in another therapeutic modality or combination of therapies.

B. The Winter Program

From year to year the specific activities that Unitas provides for children during the winter program vary somewhat, although art therapy, psychodrama, play therapy, and remedial reading are usual offerings. The winter program tends to be less recreational and more directly and individually therapeutic than the summer program, in part because of the increased numbers of trained social work staff. In the summer, little work with families takes place outside of the daytime schedule; in the winter, group therapy sessions are scheduled during both days and evenings for teens and biological families.

The extended family circle takes on a slightly different complexion during the winter. Instead of convening four days a week, it meets only once, on Thursday afternoons. Beginning at 3:15 p.m. children enter the St. Athanasius gym. Eismann greets each child at the door, making sure that each joins his or her symbolic family in the growing circle forming on the floor. Once everyone is seated, Eismann joins the circle and officially begins the meeting.

Unlike the summer program, the winter program begins with the circle and is followed by recreation time. Because it is now indoors, the circle is quieter and more orderly than it was in July and August. The substantive portion of the meeting does not change significantly from the summer, nor does the structure. The circle lasts for about one-half hour with Eismann leading the proceedings. About 4 p.m. the circle adjourns for playtime which lasts one hour.

After recreation time the circle reconvenes briefly for two purposes. It is a time to say goodbye to everyone and it is a time to have a lost-and-found service. Eismann calls on the children one by one, asking for items which they may have lost or found in the course of the afternoon. Pens, pencils, hats, and balls are exchanged with a word of thanks. Each activity, no matter how small and insignificant, has been carefully thought out and designed for its therapeutic value. In the example of the lost-and-found, the children learn about returning possessions to their rightful owners and about the style required in giving and taking. The child who does not thank the finder of a lost item receives direct and immediate disapproval from his or her peers.

At 5:30 the children leave for home, being seen to the door by their symbolic parents. The entire staff of symbolic parents, therapists, consultants, and administrators then meet for one hour to discuss therapeutic or business matters. This distinction, however is somewhat misleading since business matters often become grist for the therapeutic mill.

The following example, taken from a teen circle meeting, illustrates the blurring of business and therapeutic issues. The overarching theme of this session was the maintenance of concentration on what the therapist is doing psychodynamically. A therapist at Unitas related to the group a complaint made by the mother of a young teen who had been coming to Unitas for several years. It was early June so Unitas was making preparations for the summer program. Peter's mother complained to the therapist that her son had not heard whether his appointment to a summer job was definite. The mother expressed fear that although Peter was promised the job he would not get it, which had happened to him the year before. Eismann begins to question the therapist more closely about Peter's mother's feelings, to which the therapist, now clearly annoyed, replies, "It wasn't a therapy session. I just met her casually on the street." Unruffled, Eismann directs his questions to the rest of the group:

> What happens to make a mother go to an outside source rather than to the child? Is Peter not clear?

Several ideas are offered by different people in the group, but soon they are back to the practical issue of whether Peter is on the summer roster of teen workers and is really interested in being a summer worker. Within several minutes, however, Eismann moves the discussion away from the business issues and into the realm of psychological training.

> I want to pick up on the therapist's statement that he met Peter's mother casually on the street and that it wasn't a therapy session. Whenever we meet someone, casually or not, it is the best place. This neighborhood is our therapeutic community, hence all interactions within it are to be understood as occasions for therapeutic intervention.

These inner-circle meetings are run in the same way as the extended family circle meetings, with one predominant male leader who directs the flow of interactions and determines, to a large extent, the direction of all discussion. Generally, this person is Eismann. However, Unitas has begun to move towards the training of other individuals -- notably members of the inner-core of male workers who have been participating fully in Unitas for a number of years. These young men are receiving training with the express purpose of moving them into leadership roles within Unitas.

Like the extended family circle meetings, but on a much smaller level -- with 10 to 20 people present rather than 100 to 200 -- inner-circle meetings fulfill several purposes. They enable the staff to deal with business matters such as the tracking down of an absent teen or the scheduling of activities. A second purpose is to train the workers in therapeutic theory and techniques, as illustrated above. Third, they permit group members to express their feelings toward their work, the children, and other workers. In this respect, these meetings are peripherally therapeutic for the participants.

Built into the structure of Unitas is flexibility to adapt to the needs of the children and the workers. In Autumn 1979 several of the older teens expressed the need for more time devoted to their personal concerns, that is, time that would be explicitly therapeutic for them. There are now three such therapy groups for teenagers who meet weekly at Unitas. They all take place on Thursday evenings, after the extended family circle and inner-circle meetings and are run by either Eismann or Stekas, the Unitas administrator and social worker. The impetus for these meetings came from Stekas who had developed close relationships with the teenage girls and the college-age boys. She organized therapy sessions for each of these groups. The third group includes the remaining younger teenagers and is directed by Eismann.

C. *Staff*

Just as the organization of the Unitas program has changed through the years and continues to change even at the time of this writing, so, too, has the staff composition. The main figure who has remained constant in the history of Unitas is Eismann, although his role in Unitas is changing as he turns more responsibility over to the program administrator and the experienced workers.

The staff composition of Unitas has changed primarily in response to the funding situation of the program and the agency. From its beginning in 1968 until the present, the director of Unitas has been Edward P. Eismann, creator of the program and prime mover in its development and incorporation as an autonomous agency. During its early years, while it still functioned as a limited outreach program working out of a local community mental health center, Unitas had no full-time staff. Eismann, aided from time to time by the community mental health center staff and later by a teacher from the local elementary school and by teenagers, carried the full burden of administering, organizing, recruiting, and leading, not to mention providing therapy, the main purpose of the program.

Since its incorporation in the spring of 1977 when it began to function autonomously and receive outside financing, Unitas has expanded programming and staffing. During its first autonomous year, Unitas had, in addition to Eismann, a full-time masters-level social worker who specialized in family therapy. Also hired, for two consecutive six-month periods, were two male teenagers for Youth

Worker positions. During 1978-79 there were two B.A.-level social workers on the staff, both Puerto Rican. Their main responsibilities were to do family therapy and play therapy, although both inevitably became involved in other aspects of the program such as administrative duties and individual counseling of children. Both left within one year of arriving at Unitas, although one of them continues his relationship with Unitas. From September 1978 to May 1979 two Puerto Rican MSW students from New York University interned at Unitas, fulfilling roles similar to those of their predecessors. During this year Unitas also hired, on a per hour consultant basis, an art therapist, a remedial reading instructor, and a psychodramatist. These specialists participated only on Thursday afternoons for the extended family circle sessions during the winter program.

In January 1979 Unitas hired an MSW social worker, Lynn Stekas, to serve as full-time administrator of the agency. Through professional contacts Stekas brought in two college-level social work students to complete one-year training internships at Unitas. In October 1979, after the B.A.-level social worker and the MSW students had left, Eismann and Stekas decided to hire additional staff. Three MSW student interns from New York University began unpaid clinical training at Unitas. A full-time administrative assistant with college training in both business and psychology was also hired, as well as a secretary to tend to the agency's growing administrative needs.

D. *Teenagers and Children*

Through the years there has been a steady corps of teenage volunteers -- many of whom are paid whenever funds are available -- who have maintained the program, regardless of its financial vacillations. While full-time paid staff is a relatively new phenomenon within Unitas, these volunteer teens date back to Unitas' inception and, indeed, form an important part of the Unitas notion of therapeutic community.

During the summer of 1979, thirty teens were employed at Unitas to fill the roles of symbolic parents, aunts, and uncles. This population can be divided into three groups. First, there were uncommitted teens who worked at Unitas for the summer only, most of them referred by the Youth Employment Program. Second, there were more committed teens who had worked at Unitas before the summer program and continued to work there after the summer program ended. Third, five inner-core workers who are situated between the teen workers and the professional staff in both responsibilities and prestige. The duties of this group were more similar to those of the staff, but these teens were not hired, as was the staff, to perform a specific duty. By their own description, these teens "grew up" in Unitas and consider it an integral part of their lives. The approximate ratio of workers to children during the summer is one to seven. This ratio increases to one worker for every nine children in the winter program when more children participate in a greater variety of therapeutic activities and fewer full-time workers are available to serve them. These figures should be understood as averages since from one program piece to another the ratio can jump from one worker to several children, in art therapy, to one worker to one child, as in individual psychotherapy, to two or three workers per child, as in a crisis situation.

During the summer of 1979, teenage workers and adult staff completed questionnaires concerning various aspects of their lives. At the same time, 150 children in Unitas were interviewed. The purpose in obtaining comparative information on the children and the workers was twofold: First, such data were viewed as providing a baseline for understanding the structure and functioning of the program. A program cannot be adequately assessed without knowledge of the people it serves and the people who provide the service. Second, once these data were available, the two groups could be compared to determine demographic and socioeconomic similarities and differences.

The questionnaires filled out by the teenagers and the adult staff presented few problems. Interviews with children, however, were not as easily accomplished. Most noteworthy was the difficulty encountered in establishing the exact number of participating children. At any one time, regardless of which aspects of the program are operating fully, there are approximately 300 children active in Unitas. Exact numbers are not available, however, because participants sometimes fail to register, some have spotty attendance records, and the programs often change, for example, the summer program lasts only eight weeks. In addition, many children, because of their young age, were unable to provide adequate answers to the questions. In such cases, family members were consulted whenever possible.

The interviews were conducted with 120 of the 184 officially registered children and 30 unregistered children who were participating in the program. Sixty-four registered children were not interviewed for a variety of reasons, including: the child had left the program to visit family in Puerto Rico; the child only came to Unitas as a visitor or for a special trip; the child had stopped coming; the child was too young to answer the questions and no one was available to assist; or the child simply could not be located at the time of the interview. Each interview was conducted by one person who, in most cases, knew the child well. In all, there were ten trained interviewers, all full-time Unitas workers. The interview took about half an hour to complete.

Also during the summer of 1979, for a period of five weeks, all Unitas symbolic parents were required to keep daily attendance records of each child in his or her family. Tabulating these data as available for 120 children of the 150 who were subsequently interviewed, average attendance, out of a possible maximum of 25 meetings, was 14, producing an attendance rate of 56 percent. The rate was lower (52 percent) for children between the ages of two and nine, and higher (59 percent) for children between the ages of ten and fifteen. Children aged nine and younger averaged thirteen months at Unitas compared to the over sixteen month average of older children. For both younger and older children, however, the mode was two months, indicating that many children first entered Unitas at the start of the summer program. The longer a child has been in Unitas the better his or her attendance record. For those in the program three months or less the average attendance rate is 52 percent, while those in the program over two years have an average attendance rate of over 62 percent.

Table 1 presents selected sociobiographical characteristics of the workers and children participating in Unitas during July and August of 1979. Members of the staff and teenagers are both classified as workers since they functioned in similar ways during this period. The staff includes MSW student interns, B.A.-level social workers, and administrative personnel.

One hundred and fifty children were interviewed along with thirty-seven workers, of whom seven were senior staff -- excluding Eismann -- and thirty were teenagers. The age range of the children was from two to fourteen, with ten being the average age. The average age of the workers was nineteen.

The fact that 64 percent of the children are male is initially striking. However, this statistic is consistent with the findings of Canino *et al.*[4] that male rates of admission to psychiatric facilities are about twice as high as female rates. Thus, the percentage of males is about what should be expected. Among the teenage workers there was roughly the same predominance of males over females. In general, boys were attracted to the groups headed by males, and girls to the female-headed groups. The one exception to this pattern of male predominance was among the senior staff where five of the seven were female.

[4] Canino, Ian A., Brian F. Earley, and Lloyd H. Rogler. *The Puerto Rican Child in New York City: Stress and Mental Health*, Monograph No. 4, Hispanic Research Center, Fordham University, Bronx, New York, 1980.

TABLE 1
Selected Sociobiographical Characteristics of Workers and Children in Unitas, Summer 1979

Characteristics	Workers	Children
Mean age (years)	19	10
Sex (%)		
Male	60	64
Female	40	36
Education (%)		
In school	73	96
Out of school	22	4
Not available	5	--
Last grade completed (mean, in years)	12	4
Ethnicity (%)		
Hispanic	68	91
Black	27	7
Other	5	2
Religion (%)		
Catholic	54	51
Protestant	32	26
Other	14	23
Language spoken at home (%)		
Mostly English	46	19
Mixed	43	34
Mostly Spanish	11	47
Family structure (%)		
One-parent family	41	47
Other	59	53

Since about half the children are referred to Unitas by schools, it is not surprising that levels of educational participation are high. In fact, all children of school age were attending school. The percentage of workers in school is obviously reduced by the senior staff, most of whom have completed school. Among the teenagers, one-half of those who graduated from high school in June 1980 entered college the following September.

The majority of both workers and children were Hispanics, most of whom identified themselves as Puerto Ricans. The advantages of cultural affinity in the Unitas program are quite obvious. In this context, the larger proportion of blacks among the workers is interesting and, possibly, significant.

The religious backgrounds of workers and children are very similar. The high percentage of Catholics is to be expected in an Hispanic population. However, the number of children in the "other" category is much higher because about 12 percent did not know what, if any, their religious affiliations were. Similar religious background, like similar cultural background, may be valuable in promoting worker-child compatibility.

Although Spanish is the language most often used in the home, particularly among the children, English is the language spoken at Unitas. While this practical bilingualism is well known among those who work with or study Hispanic children, its cultural and psychological implications are important. This characteristic needs to be viewed in relation to its effect on the child.

In family structure, both the children and the workers have a high percentage of one-parent families. While these figures are high, they are consistent with those of the general Puerto Rican population of New York City where about 39 percent of all Puerto Rican households are headed by single parents.[5] As will be evident later in this study, the Unitas program is specifically designed to cope with this situation.

In general, the table reveals that the characteristics of the children and the workers are very similar. Not only are the key factors of language and culture fairly close, but also religious affiliation and family structure are similar. Since the majority of authority figures that the children see, in terms of doctors, teachers, police, television personalities and others, would not be culturally similar, this affinity between Unitas worker and child very likely is useful both for enhancing communication and ethnic pride.

The theme which integrates the various aspects of the Unitas program is the importance of the family and the relationships

[5] National Puerto Rican Forum, *The Next Step Toward Equality: A Comprehensive Study of Puerto Ricans in the United States Mainland*. New York, 1980, p. 10.

between family members. In Unitas families, as in real families, such relationships are often difficult, involving love, interdependence, closeness, and trust. By focusing the Unitas family on these positive concepts and needs, teaching how to communicate effectively with others, without violence, Unitas blurs the distinctions between mental health and mental illness, a term which one rarely hears from Unitas workers. The philosophy which underlies the workings of Unitas -- from its organization to its therapeutic techniques -- forms the basis of the following chapter.

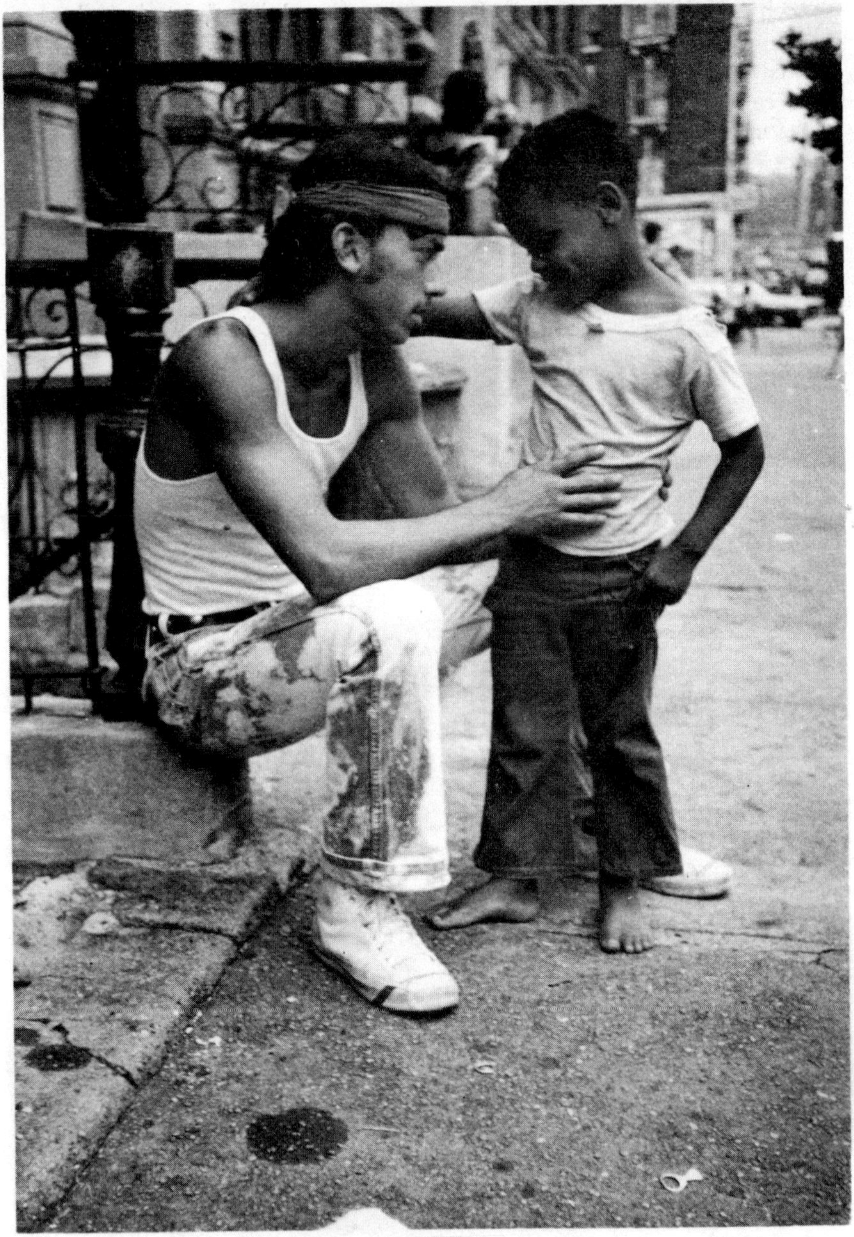

PLATE 3. The essence of healing resides in the energy of love that is communicated and responded to by the other.

II

PHILOSOPHY OF HEALING

We meet together to help each other.
We meet together to care for each other.
We meet together to control each other.
We meet together to share our thoughts and our hearts.
This is Unitas. We are one big family
made up of little families.

With these words Eismann begins an extended family circle meeting of Unitas. The family provides a recognized symbol around which the Unitas Therapeutic Community has developed much of its philosophy and programming. For Unitas, the family is a highly emotional, potentially powerful therapeutic structure in which individuals learn to bond with one another. It is through the family -- both real and symbolic -- that Unitas teaches the troubled youth of the South Bronx about the range of human emotions and interactions.

The family, as an ideal structure, is the symbol of the Unitas therapeutic group. Every teenager and child can readily identify as a son or daughter, sister or brother, from first-hand experience with parents and siblings. By relating to others in Unitas according to these familiar kinship statuses they gain an understanding of the problems of interaction within a family and learn ways of resolving them. As Eismann points out, it is the responsibility of the entire group to handle conflict.

Unitas justifies this approach to children through both real and symbolic family systems on psychological grounds. Eismann writes that through the years:

> Unitas had become a symbolic family where youth were often helped to get from each other what they

> were often lacking in whole or in part in their actual family lives, which lack was theorized to result in behavioral or symptomatic disabilities. This lack was seen as essentially the absence of one or two experiences or both: a lack of positive group belonging and at least one deeply felt nurturing friendship with someone else, regardless of age or sex. Without these two provisions, maladjustment was seen as highly likely. The experience of positive group belonging was understood as ordinarily provided to a child by his biological family unit and the deeply felt nurturing friendship as ordinarily provided by nurturing parents or parent substitute. But for the troubled child where family life is usually so dysfunctional and its rehabilitation so questionable, an alternative symbolic family care system was created by Unitas in which provision for emotional care of children was developed and built into the local neighborhood network. This "family care" system was seen as best offered through the therapeutic community concept.

The Unitas method is not one of psychotherapy as, for example, psychoanalysis, although it propounds certain methods and philosophies of therapy more than others. Unitas is an enterprise whose goal is psychological healing. Such healing, according to Eismann, may be effected through a broad variety of approaches which aim to restore wholeness to body, mind, and spirit. Conceptually, the broader term "healing" refers to all those actions which aim to establish or re-establish well-being to the whole person, not necessarily focused exclusively on the psyche. In its approach to the whole person, Unitas also aims to provide an environment for the children which is clean, orderly and pollution-free (no smoking, drugs, and unnecessary noise), and encourages a health orientation which includes exercise, good nutritional practices, and physical touch. While such holistic approaches and concepts are recognized and supported within the overall orientation to healing, it is primarily in the interpersonal components of psychological healing that Unitas concentrates its strongest practice. These interpersonal methodologies can be reduced to two: therapeutic community and psychotherapy.

A. *Therapeutic Community as Healing*

Therapeutic community, as contrasted with psychotherapy, is a form of *milieu* therapy which stresses the importance of cultivating a positive, cooperative, mutually helpful and encouraging interpersonal environment within the context of an educative or treatment setting.

Eismann gives central importance to a modified version of the therapeutic community paradigm frequently used in mental hospitals. This model, originally explicated by Maxwell Jones, describes the therapeutic community as follows:

> The therapeutic community is distinctive among other comparable treatment centres in the way the institution's total resources, both staff and patients, are self-consciously pooled in furthering treatment. This implies above all a change in the usual status of patients. In collaboration with the staff, they now become active participants in the therapy of other patients and in other aspects of overall hospital work -- in contrast to their relatively more passive recipient role in conventional treatment regimes.[6]

There are three principal lines of social interaction within a therapeutic community: the patient and his peers; the patient and the doctor; and the patient and the junioi nursing staff. Jones advocates the development of these communication networks and their integration into the coherent treatment of the patients.[7] With the opening of these channels there is an increase of patient participation in his or her own and other patients' treatment, in ward administration, and in the use of community and group treatment. There is also a concomitant decrease in individual psychotherapy. Such changes result in a shift in the social organization of the ward "from a predominantly hierarchical one...in the direction of a democratic, equalitarian one."[8] As patients assume greater responsibilities in their own treatment and that of other patients their roles gradually become closer to those of the staff. According to Jones, these changes lead to the acceptance of new values and cultural concepts.

Although originally developed for use in the organization of a psychiatric unit of a hospital, the therapeutic community concept has been applied to other treatment settings. Indeed, Jones recognized such possibilities, writing that

[6] Jones, Maxwell. "Towards a Clarification of the 'Therapeutic Community' Concept." In Rossi, Jean J. and William J. Filstead (eds.), *The Therapeutic Community*. New York: Behavioral Publications, 1973, p. 17.

[7] *Ibid.*, p. 19.

[8] *Ibid.*, p. 22.

> The original descriptions of therapeutic communities were usually within the structure of a psychiatric facility, generally a hospital. But with the growth of community psychiatric ideas, the system has moved in the direction of extra hospital settings, such as the community mental health center, a drop-in clinic, or out-patient department situated in the neighborhood of the patient's home. Even closer to the patient's or potential patient's home environment is the home visit for assessment purposes, and the development of a treatment programme involving the patient's own family, or extended family system, and often operating within his immediate home environment. Thus there has been a continuous trend from the artificial setting of the hospital to a much closer involvement with the social casualty in his real-life setting.[9]

Eismann borrowed some characteristics of Jones' therapeutic community and adapted them for use with children and adolescents in the South Bronx. The principles, practices, and common organizational elements guiding the operation of a therapeutic community and the modifications introduced to Unitas are described below.

First, the therapeutic community concept, originally developed for use within an institutional framework, removed from normal life, proposes that close contact be maintained between the program and the community outside the institutional setting. Operating within the institution, usually a hospital, the treatment program, to be consistent with the philosophy, needed explicitly to formulate ways to assure contact with real life outside the institution. Unitas does not remove the child from his native social environment and does not, therefore, face such a problem. Eismann refers to Bleuler's recognition of the limitations of the institution in treating patients:

> The institution as such does not cure the disease. However, it may be valuable from an educational viewpoint, it may alleviate acute, agitated states due to psychic influences. At the same time it carries with it the danger that the patient may become too estranged from normal life and also that the relatives get accustomed to the idea of the institution. In

[9] *Ibid.*, p. 325.

general, it is preferable to treat these patients under their usual conditions and within their usual surroundings.[10]

Eismann describes the treatment setting of Unitas to illustrate how the program has modified the therapeutic community concept:

> The treatment setting is the neighborhood street itself, local school, local community center, local church center -- all familiar social environments for the child. There is no emphasis on treatment within hospital, clinic, or "special school" structures. It is virtually impossible to build real life experiences and responses within institutional frameworks removed from actual living.

If the desirable therapeutic setting should be as close as possible to the natural environment of the patient, Unitas, then, treats patients in their true natural social *milieu.*

Second, a therapeutic community within a hospital is not to be confused with the functioning of the hospital itself, which houses and administers the community. In contrast, the administrative component of Unitas is virtually continuous with the community itself. The patient who goes to a mental health clinic or hospital does not become a member of the institution. But when a child comes to Unitas, he or she is not merely a recipient of services but a member who belongs, as to a church, a fraternity, a patriotic organization, a tribe, a family. It may be argued that such is the nature of a hospital therapeutic community or even group therapy. What is significant in Unitas is the intensity and extent of the bonding that takes place and the loyalty that results, because of both its ties within the neighborhood community and those that it creates within itself and among the children.

Some of the participants in Unitas -- usually older teens or young adults who have spent many years in the program -- are conscious of these bonds of loyalty, founded on utmost devotion in exchange for receiving honor, privileges, status, friendship, and support. Other participants may have only a dim sense of Unitas as an entity apart from the many fragments of it in which they take part. They may only understand Eismann's teachings and exhortations during family circle meetings in a very literal way. For

[10] Bleuler, E. *Dementia Precox or the Group of Schizophrenia.* New York: International Universities Press, 1950, p. 328. Quoted in Ozarin, Ludy D. "Moral Treatment and the Mental Hospital" in Rossi, Jean J. and William J. Filstead (eds.), *The Therapeutic Community.* New York: Behavioral Publications, 1973, pp. 29-46.

example, they know that they have to be at a certain place at a certain time, that they must seat themselves in a certain way, that there are prescribed methods of making their wants known, of addressing the group, of calling for silence or attention. Such spatial, temporal, and behavioral markers and boundaries, in combination with a regular cast of participants, provide a structure which children may internalize for therapeutic benefit.

Third, the population being treated within the traditional therapeutic community which Jones describes is psychologically different from the population treated within Unitas. Patients generally enter a hospital setting for treatment through professional referrals. They are admitted by a physician in charge and then referred to a unit psychiatrist. Patients then become part of a therapeutic community made up entirely of other patients with symptomatologies almost identical or similar to their own. It is not expected that psychologically "normal" individuals will be found as patients within this context.

In Unitas,

> ...there is no separation of disturbed and "normal" children. The influence of healthy children on problem children is the therapeutic wedge. The power of healing resides in the healthy segments of the organism; that is, the natural social network.

This mingling of disturbed and healthy children finds reinforcement in the Unitas referral system. Children enter Unitas through a variety of networks: a school guidance counselor, the child's parent or other relative, a friend already in Unitas, a Unitas worker, or through personal interest. Some children, watching the program in action from the tenement windows during the summer, find themselves lured into participating. The children who require more intensive treatment receive it, individually within their biological family or within a peer group. Regardless of the treatment modes used, virtually all children attend the weekly Unitas circle meetings. Here there is no distinction made between troubled and healthy children either in the symbolic families in which they choose to participate or in their manner of treatment by workers and peers. Eismann writes:

> The symbolic family and the one-to-one needed relationships are built naturally into children's lives. There is no identification of children as mentally sick either by themselves or others, which identification would lead to further dehumanization. People are merely people with the feelings of any one human being echoed in some way in every other human being.

In addition, Unitas offers a structural flexibility which facilitates openness of expression and freedom of movement, as one would find in a true "outside" community. Since there is no formal admitting procedure comparable to that of a hospital and no formal discharge procedure, children are obliged to set the boundaries of their own participation and that of their fellows. Although a minority of children participate only sporadically, most children stay in the program for at least one year. In 1979, the average time spent in Unitas by children, aged 15 and under, was 13.6 months and this figure is a conservative one since it does not include teen workers, many of whom have been in Unitas for much longer.

Fourth, the traditional therapeutic community focuses only on the treatment of mental disorder, neglecting prevention, a logical result of the fact that healthy individuals are excluded from participation. Unitas, integrating healthy and problem children within its therapeutic system, deals with both treatment and prevention on primary, secondary, and tertiary levels.

> Treatment and prevention go hand in hand. As a community system heals its problems (in place of cutting them off) or prevents them from developing in the first place, it reinforces its health. It is a form of "inoculation" against future disease.

Fifth, in a therapeutic community the patient is conceptualized as an active agent in treatment. Unitas builds on this notion, training teenagers as psychological caretakers for younger children. Moreover, in its teachings, all are viewed as dependent on and responsible for their neighbors and themselves. Helping takes place not only when an outside professional intervenes in an interaction, but also when ordinary people reach out to understand and care for one another.

Sixth, there is an effort made in a therapeutic community to flatten the traditional two-class system of staff and patients in order to create a sense of unity. In Unitas, the traditional split between staff and patients is blurred by the intermediate teenage group which functions in both capacities. However, the program maintains a strict hierarchy for psychotherapeutic purposes, which distinguishes clearly and significantly between symbolic grandfather, parents, aunts and uncles, older children, and younger children. Even with these structural constraints, Unitas succeeds in giving its participants responsibility for the operation and governing of the program and involving them in administrative and therapeutic decision-making.

Seventh, the therapeutic community fosters open and direct communication between staff and patients. Such communication is an explicit intermediate goal of Unitas, necessary to achieve the higher goals of psychological and social mental well-being and human interdependence.

Finally, the scheduling of frequent, regular meetings in which all members of the community participate as part of the patient's treatment characterizes the running of a therapeutic community. In addition to formal social and therapeutic groups, informal and unplanned group situations become important parts of patient psychotherapy. Unitas relies on frequent formal and informal group meetings for its functioning. Throughout the year, especially during the summer, all the children, teenagers and staff meet formally in the extended family circle. Smaller groups with more specific goals and membership meet in the teenage circle, teenage support groups, art therapy groups, remedial reading groups, and play therapy groups. Teenagers and children meet informally in their natural settings -- home, street, school -- and in Unitas during unstructured free time set aside for relaxed interactions.

B. *Psychotherapy as Healing*

Eismann defines psychotherapy as "an educational process rather than a medical transaction." He explains that it is

> ...a systematic way of dealing with emotional and mental problems through psychological means, to heal the hurt. In therapy there is a carefully designed plan of intervention involving a way of understanding the problem that gave rise to the symptom. If it's understood that Peter is depressed, there's a psychological understanding that he might be furious and has "swallowed his own rage," or that he is overcome with a feeling of profound discouragement. Eliciting rage or voicing the discouragement is not itself the cure of the symptom. An understanding of the purpose of the symptom and addressing this purpose in an empathic re-educative manner are even more importantly the plan in psychotherapeutic practice.

The goal of psychotherapy is

> ...to enable people to become psychically comfortable and reasonably responsible in their work, their relationships and their attitude toward life...so that the person becomes master over his thoughts and

> feelings, owning up to them responsibly. We are helping the person's ideas about living to expand so that he can consider other points of view and modify his own restricted perceptions. When distorted perceptions are "healed" through therapy, psychic energy, heretofore locked into one's neurosis or psychosis, is freed to use in real living.

While the therapeutic community concept aims to remediate and prevent dysfunctional behavior on a broad scale by maintaining the *milieu* necessary for healing relationships to be experienced by all in similar fashion, the psychotherapies focus more precisely on diagnosed mental stress areas. Thus, psychotherapy aims to effect a healing of broken interpersonal relationships, particularly of ones past but manifested in the present. Broken interpersonal relationships constitute the mental stress areas that psychotherapy in Unitas aims at healing specifically. In this kind of psychological healing, there is a deliberate use of psychological interventions based on scientific or pseudo-scientific rationales, usually derived from psychoanalytic theory, and of specific plans of action designed to heal distortions or brokenness of the mind.

Since in addition to the therapeutic community, psychotherapy is the primary approach used in Unitas to effect its goal of psychological healing, it is important to understand how this is understood and practiced in Unitas.

Above, Eismann described psychotherapy essentially as a systematic way of understanding and dealing with emotional hurts in an empathic re-educative manner. He emphasized the correction of distorted perceptions through the therapeutic relationship, thereby enabling a person to relate more productively to people, work, and life as a whole. Although Eismann speaks of re-education and the correction of distorted perceptions as essential components of psychotherapy, he appears to give these activities second place to the relationship component. Indeed, Unitas places extreme emphasis on the relationship component, whether or not insight or re-education ever takes place. It is through the experience of love in the relationship that healing may or may not miss its mark, depending on the love component. The essence of psychotherapy resides in the energy of love that is communicated and responded to by the other. This love is a force - conceived of as psychological, psychic, and spiritual - which has intrinsically psychological effects. Its transmission to another generates something life-giving, a healing to some felt brokenness. Love, however, can occur independently of psychotherapy as a plan of action by itself. It follows, then, that the healer need not be a therapist formally trained in certain techniques, with a particular body of knowledge and an understanding of the genesis of the problem. Healing forces are possessed by all people as certain "qualities, dispositions, or gifts" such as the power to love, to have faith and hope. Therefore, we must not necessarily assume that a therapist is an effective healer for everyone or for all problems.

Eismann speaks of this healing force as the "charisma of love," a power each person has, some more, some less, to influence or touch the minds and hearts of others. This love can be intellectually or poetically defined, as it has been by scholars, artists, and psychoanalytic practitioners, becoming thereby subjective, elusive, limited, and even contradictory. Eismann prefers to speak of the characteristics or "fruits" of love, expressed through the effects of a healing relationship.

> It is through a special kind of relationship that the charisma of love energizes and heals the brokenness of others. Love is an attentiveness that listens empathically; inspires and communicates faith and hope because it has this belief in the strength and goodness of another, touched by it and responding to it; accepts and allows another to feel what they feel without external or internal criticism and judgment; encourages the movement of growth though not where one might choose to grow oneself; has a passionate involvement and faith in the process of healing, in general, and pointedly the specific person one is to heal; experiences a close, warm feeling toward the other, but with an unpossessive love; is able to transmit all the foregoing with an authentic realness. Love is also much that is unspoken and subliminal.

Eismann describes his concept of love as "an integration of Biblical, Buberian, Rogerian, Adlerian, and psychoanalytical thinking." It is an experiential love that heals, one that aims at correcting the arrests and fixations of the past as well as the losses and traumas of the present. It is precisely the deprivation of love, especially in childhood, that emotional distress and mental disorders reflect. The greater a person's deprivation of parenting love, the deeper the level of substitute parenting he needs in a relationship to become whole. Eismann stresses that theories of experiential psychotherapy demand this type of symbolic parenting with its nurturing love, but frequently such a demand frightens a healer, so he may find himself, in the name of therapeutic neutrality, withdrawing from the very feelings he should be using in healing. Yet, Eismann points out that the literature explicitly demands that

> ...the therapist should enter into communion with

> the one to be healed; there should be empathy between the two and the healer should love the person. Properly understood, loving another in need of healing, in the sense described, may be the one thing decisively therapeutic to the person in need. This "Buberian" relatedness is an absolute requirement. The question raised is: "Is love, as described, enough?" If the love is empathic on needed levels, is not possessive or exploitive and is genuine, probably it is enough, but it is a controversial point. For the children and families we work with in Unitas it may be enough since we are dealing with multi-problem, character-disordered, borderline type personalities as well as with neglected and abused children. The corrective emotional experience or re-parenting, using a developmental model as a framework, appears to bring about most of the behavioral changes we witness. I call it "holding children's hands as they are growing up."

Eismann points out in this regard that studies of individual, family, and group treatment demonstrate that warmth, empathy, and genuiness have been found necessary if not sufficient in themselves to help people change.

Eismann is not arguing against therapies that stress interpretation or insight. He comments that "through the kind of communion that evolves in a loving relationship, insights naturally flow and can be consciously surfaced by a skilled healer." It is at this point in therapy that emotional re-education at a cognitive level can be effected. Eismann's stress on the essential power of love to heal is born of his understanding of the literature on healing, his own experience in the flowering of Unitas, and his own individual and group analysis where he says insight was secondary to the impact of a relationship in bringing out his own "dormant charisma."

Eismann studied under Papanek, an Adlerian who stressed a mental health perspective and therapy that emphasized interpersonal relatedness, interdependence, and social interest. Describing the similarity between *milieu* therapy and group therapy, Eismann quotes Papanek:

> My point is that insight is of no avail where there is no healing relationship from which the insight springs and that there are many cases where the relationship alone can engender change without the aid of insight. Unless this is understood, therapists may give up too soon on patients who, for a variety of

> reasons, such as sociocultural background, education, and personal inclinations, are not prone to respond to intellectual interpretations and are unable to gain insight into their neurotic behavior patterns ...Just as patients improve in individual psychotherapy with or without insight so long as a healing relationship is operative, so, too, patients may improve even more in group therapy with or without insight through the medium of the healing *milieu* provided by the group structure and the regulating activities of the therapist.[11]

So, it is Eismann's belief, communicated throughout the system of Unitas, that it is through the loving relationships within it that healing is given and taken. He quotes Gordon Hamilton, one of the original pioneers in social work education and practice:

> Change in feeling can result from a major experience such as a happy marriage, through great physical or mental suffering, through a significant relationship with one or more persons, or through religious experience...So far as we know, it is only by means of a deeply felt experience in a relationship that treatment can affect a person's attitudes towards himself and his fellows.[12]

With his Adlerian frame of reference, it is not difficult to understand the theoretical and operational direction Eismann took in creating a mental health program aimed at family repair, the creation of symbolic families, and networking. Dealing with a child in the context of his social network, particularly his family, is basic to Adlerian practice. Over time, Unitas has adopted a family-focused interpersonal orientation to healing, reflecting the inherent capacity or charisma of healing in all people, particularly those already bonded in family or friendship networks.

As Eismann expanded his own thinking and began to draw upon the healing forces in children's natural networks, it was logical for him to turn to systems theory in general and to family therapy in particular. Many of the techniques Eismann uses in large circle groups, classrooms, and smaller groups are obviously drawn from family therapy practice, particularly from the thinking of Satir,

[11] Papanek, Helene, "Psychotherapy Without Insight: Group Therapy as Milieu Therapy." *Journal of Individual Psychology*, Vol. 17, Nov. 1961, pp. 184-192.

[12] Hamilton, Gordon, *Theory and Practice of Social Casework*. New York: Columbia University Press, 1956.

Minuchin, and Haley.[13] Extended family circle sessions are replete with family communications theory skills in which Eismann, building on Satir's thinking, focuses on maintaining an open system of dialogue in order to help children experience clear, direct, and congruent communication. Influences from outside sources are welcomed and rules can be negotiated, in contrast to the closed authoritarian systems in which physical and psychological forces operate to impede co-responsibility and co-creativity.

Eismann's views of family structure with himself as grandfather, older teens as parents, children as older and younger siblings, together with their clearly formulated hierarchical lines, are a base of operation through which support networks on all levels are maintained and tasks are prescribed. In keeping with such a structural approach to the symbolic family, echoing Minuchin and Haley, Eismann consistently changes the structure of individual symbolic families to bring influential symbolic relatives from one family to come to bear on children in other families which have not been able to heal their own members. Eismann says he often does this in real family therapy when it is evident that an acting-out youngster, for example, may respond to the interest and attention of an admired uncle. In that case, Eismann will direct the boy's mother to occupy herself with her well-behaved but friendless daughter and leave the son's management to the uncle who by this time has also been included in the family sessions.

In addition to reworking the structures of the symbolic family groupings, task assignments, and maintaining an open system of dialogue between family members, Eismann encourages the strengthening of positive bonds through empathic statements, building commonalities among the children, paraphrasing communications, and, above all, reframing all communications in such a way that defensiveness is neutralized and the positive forces of healing are released. For much of this, he is indebted to the family therapists.

When it comes to diagnosis, again Eismann thinks in family therapy systems, particularly the concept of reframing. Traditional diagnosis, according to Eismann, assumes a negative attitude toward patients and their "diseases."

[13] Satir, Virginia. *Conjoint Family Therapy*. Palo Alto, Ca.: Science and Behavior Books, 1964.

Minuchin, Salvador. *Families and Family Therapy*. Cambridge, Mass.: Harvard University Press, 1974.

Haley, Jay. *Changing Families: A Family Therapy Reader*. New York: Grune and Stratton, 1971.

> The way we phrase things determines the way we see a person. Saying "vulnerability" instead of "pathology" is a way of reframing; I do this with my workers; it is what I would do in therapy...to tap into the healthy forces of people, reframe what they say in order for them to be able to more comfortably talk about their concerns, releasing their positive energies. Pathology, being negativistic, is part of the Freudian tradition. No wonder Freud spoke so much about dealing with resistance. He helped encourage it.

Eismann stresses that therapy should "begin where the child is at." This does not, however, preclude gathering background information about the child's current life and his experiences. In order to control and direct the kind of information collected, Unitas has developed a detailed form, the "Comprehensive Clinical Assessment of Children." It covers basic information about the child, a statement of the child's problem, his psychological and medical developmental history, his school performance and his family background and structure. The form is not a schedule for asking questions, but a suggested outline of the type of information the mental health worker should keep in mind. The information is not collected in one formal intake interview but over a period of time. Explains Eismann:

> There is no distinction made between diagnosis and treatment; it is an ongoing process. There is no diagnostic intake interview in terms of presenting the client with an onslaught of prescribed questions. We try to be sensitive to our healing focus from the very beginning.

Eismann offers an example of how this philosophy of looking at the positive in a person and in a situation finds translation in everyday activities.

One day, during the summer, a group of mothers of some of the more disturbed children in Unitas happened to come to the street during play time. They began to jump rope together, not with their children, and from all accounts, were having a wonderful time. Strict Freudian thinking, according to Eismann, might interpret the behavior of these women as indicative of their ego regression, thereby placing a negative interpretation on their play. Eismann's interpretation of this event, while not ignoring the former perception, focused on the pleasure these women were deriving from their play and the company of their peers. He perceived the event as reflective of social interest and creative spontaneity. The therapist who witnessed this activity in fact viewed the situation in just this way, encouraging the women to continue. Also, seeing this as an excellent opportunity to begin interacting with these women, she briefly entered their game, which enabled the energies of bonding to take place naturally.

In concluding this section on the philosophical underpinnings of Unitas' teaching methods, theological influences are clearly integrated with the psychological and sociological influences already delineated. Although formal religion plays no explicit role in Unitas, basic Christian notions of love and interdependence find voice. In an address to clergy and laity at the Pastoral Institute of St. Joseph's Seminary at Dunwoodie, New York, in 1976, Eismann related the goals and methods of the ministry to those of Unitas:

> The question for the ministry is this: How are people led most effectively to become loving parts of each other? The model of ministry I propose is reminiscent of the early Church. It is a shared ministry with emphasis put on the entire Christian community being ministers of God's love (and thus His grace) to each other.
>
> Every Christian, indeed, every person possesses the charisma of love. It is a given as hunger is a given. For the Christian, the natural charisma of love becomes a specially consecrated power through the grace of Baptism. Through this charisma the people of God become channels of grace to each other.
>
> To build a charismatic community of love first requires the presence of potentiality for love.
>
> ...The more love is understood by any one person, the more possibilities that person has to energize the latent charismatic powers of healing in others. Psychology (particularly psychoanalytic theory) has given us profound insights into the nature of love, the effects of love on people and the effects of deprivation of love. Use of psychological thinking in creating and maintaining a community of love is a profound way of incarnating God's presence.
>
> ...In sum, where you find love shared among

a community of people, you have God's presence, and that's ministry.

Eismann, who at one time studied to become a Catholic priest, has a strong belief in Christian values and in the universal need and capacity for healing and love; therefore, whether it be called ministry or healing community, it comes as no surprise that religious elements and themes are identifiable in Unitas.

C. *Underlying Values of Unitas*

At the basis of healing -- instilling hope and faith in the people -- lies love, an overarching value which Eismann uses to encompass a number of other values which express the most positive forms of human interdependence. These values include: nurturance of the positive, i.e., the healthy parts of others; acknowledgement of the reality of one's own and others' feelings; empathy; and openness and directness of interpersonal communication. These values readily translate into technical principles and skills which Unitas teaches and fosters in its children and caretakers. Each value requires sensitivity to the needs of others and a desire to understand what the other person experiences.

The values of which Eismann speaks come closest to Adler's concept of *Gemeinschaftsgefuhl*, translated loosely as social interest or feeling. Adler writes:

> It is almost impossible to exaggerate the value of an increase in social feeling. The mind improves, for intelligence is a communal function. The feeling of worth and value is heightened, giving courage and an optimistic view, and there is a sense of acquiescence in the common advantages and drawbacks of our lot. The individual feels at home in life and feels his existence to be worthwhile just so far as he is useful to others and is overcoming common, instead of private, feelings of inferiority. Not only the ethical nature, but the right attitude in aesthetics, the best understanding of the beautiful and the ugly, will always be founded upon the truest social feeling.[14]

[14] Ansbacher, Heinz and Rowenna (eds.). *The Individual Psychology of Alfred Adler*. New York: Harper and Row, 1964, p. 155.

The focus on the positive or healthy parts of others is an aspect of the Unitas philosophy which Eismann claims sets Unitas apart from many mental health approaches following a medical model with emphasis on pathology. Eismann considers the psychiatric profession to perpetuate an error by understanding troubled children as "emotionally sick" and in need of psychiatric care. Backing up his point of view with his Adlerian frame of reference, Eismann quotes Dreikurs, a leading exponent of Adlerian psychology and group therapy:

> A new professional discipline has emerged: child psychiatry. It is based on an assumption we cannot share, that children who need help are "emotionally sick." Few of them are really sick; most are misguided. Who is most qualified to help them? The teacher, the parent, the counselor, the psychiatrist, the social worker, or any adult friend or relative. In our experience, any one of them can be effective in influencing the child and in helping him adjust. The disturbed child has wrong ideas about himself and life and uses socially unacceptable means to find his place. Everyone who can win his confidence, who understands him, who can show him alternatives, can redirect the child.[15]

Unitas stresses, above all, the inherent value of interdependence, a universal good. The need of the individual for the group and of the group for the individual is recognized, reinforced, celebrated, and promoted explicitly and implicitly within the program. The Unitas brand of interdependence emphasizes individuality within the group context with each person responsible for not only his or her own welfare but also that of others. This responsibility for others carries with it the difficult task of fostering their strengths, enabling them to function wholly in their lives. Social life can be conceptualized, then, as the interplay between the forces of self-interest and concern for others, an interplay within polarities which are constantly engaged and balanced for the survival of both the group and the individual.

Mutual dependence does not mean that members take over each other's functions. Thus, no member is to talk for or act for any other member. Unitas puts it this way: Help your brother to do it for himself. To "help" the other person, to the extent that his own

[15] Dreikurs, Rudolph. *Psychology in the Classroom*. New York: Harper and Row, 1968, p. ix.

capacities for self-care and for caring for others would atrophy, would destroy the other person as an individual with a distinct identity. The other person, thus deprived of autonomy and individuality, becomes incapable of helping others and, therefore, has not really been helped at all. The two polarities -- the individual and the group -- cannot always harmonize, however, since individual needs may run counter to group needs at any moment in the ongoing interaction. While the aim of Unitas is to promote the mental health of the individual child, the preferred means for doing this involve activation of the group or community. The uppermost aim then is to maintain group functioning in a process which will provide a sense of belonging for the children. The individual, thus, becomes subordinated to the group for his or her own welfare. We come full circle when we realize that this interdependence is based essentially on the belief that people can heal one another through their charisma or gift of healing.

An example of a way this interdependence is fostered on a one-to-one level, with repercussions on the group level, is through the pairing of troubled children with teenage caretakers. Raul, a 14-year old who has been in Unitas for a little over a year, lives two doors away from David, a troubled 10-year old. Eismann determined that David, one of the more disruptive and needy children in Unitas, would benefit from frequent gentle contact with an "older" male figure. Linking David with Raul, who is closely supervised by Eismann and supported by other teens and trained staff, appeared to be a solution. Raul is encouraged to check in on David every day, to play with him after school, bring him food, engage him in a variety of activities in a one-to-one relationship in order to promote bonding between himself and the boy. No pressure is placed on David to deal with his problems; rather he is learning first that he has a friend in Raul, someone he can turn to if there is a problem. Raul talks of how frustrating it is to work with David and how he tires of reaching out to him only to be repeatedly rejected. The teen group in which Raul participates (made up of symbolic mothers and fathers) steps in to help Raul figure out his own and David's needs. After lengthy discussion, Raul feels encouraged to continue with David, recognizing both the strides David has made and the difficulties being faced. Raul is growing from his experience with David and with the group while David benefits from his interactions with Raul. The group of teenagers also profits in learning how to help Raul, and feel closer to him. Eismann often points out how satisfying it can be to make a connection with another person, to feel that you have been able to help that individual move forward in his or her life.

Finally, handmaiden to the values of love, interdependence, and individuation within the group context is the value of mastery. Mastery, achievement in the sense of control in the individual, artistic, or physical realms (including athletics, dance, or physical fitness), is emphasized as a means to foster the more basic values. Mastery of the interpersonal aspects of life -- constructively open communication, effective give-and-take of emotional and material supplies, and caring for each other and for oneself within the interpersonal context -- is the primary goal. It is through a control over one's world -- whether through learning to tumble on the mats or to speak up in a group of peers -- that the child begins to gain self-confidence, necessary to be a whole person relating to others. Eismann's view is that a child's lack of mastery -- of interpersonal or materially-based skills -- is a sign of his more basic psychological deprivation. The gaining of a sense of mastery, then, becomes a way for children to have positive experiences in relation to others, as they gain, too, a sense of belonging to a caring group.

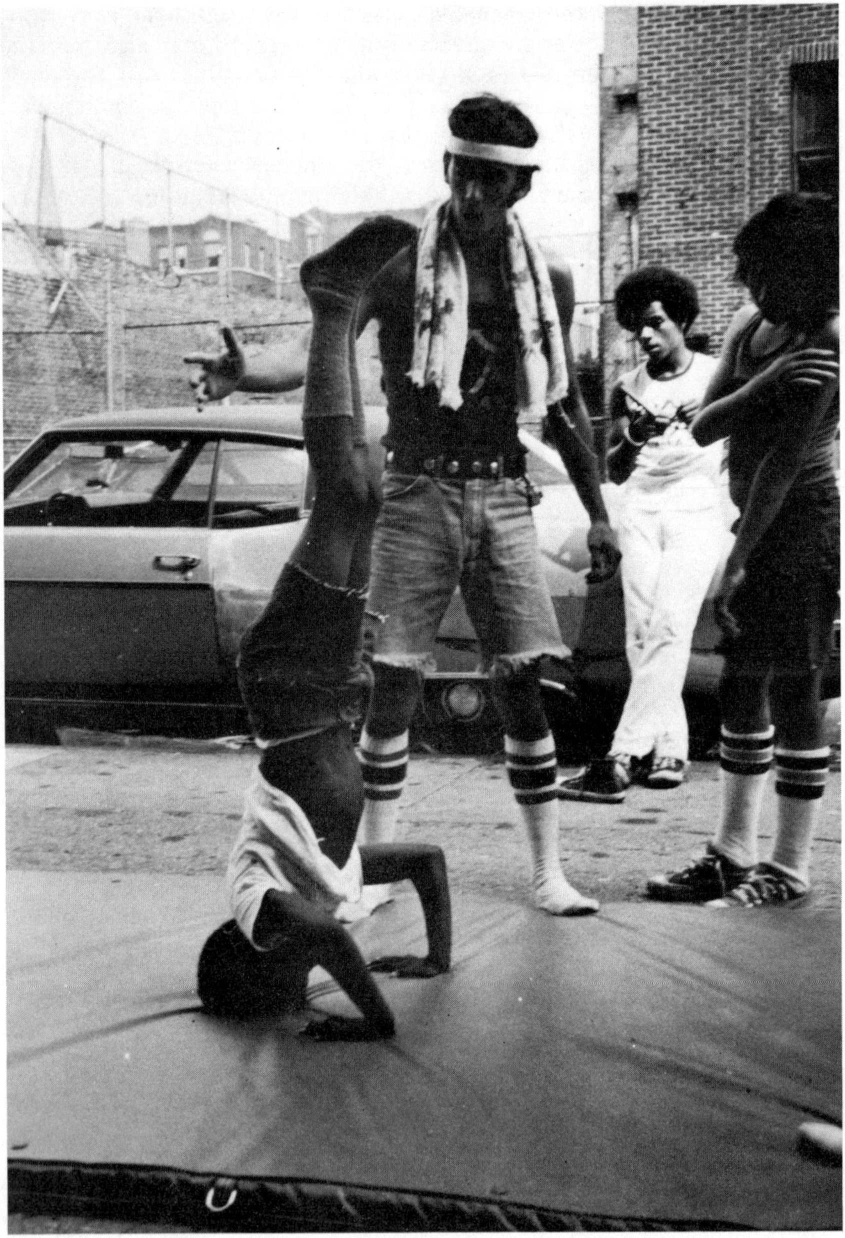

PLATE 4. Autonomy: not independence but interdependence . . . to stand on one's own with a helping hand if needed.

III

HEALING MODALITIES AND TECHNIQUES

In the previous chapter we described the philosophical background of Unitas' concept of a healing force imbedded in human relationships. This section discusses how healing takes place; that is, the specific therapeutic systems and techniques developed by Unitas to treat its children. Vital to the understanding of the healing process is the importance of the family as both a symbol of healing and a vehicle for bringing it about.

A. *The Extended Family Circle as Community Therapy*

The extended family circle is the one therapeutic mode of Unitas which brings together its philosophy, its therapeutic techniques, and all its children, teenagers, and staff. The extended family circle also dramatizes the social structure of Unitas, clearly revealing its hierarchy of authority. In the family circle two symbolic systems are combined: the family and ritual, the former becoming the base which is manipulated and played upon by the latter.

Family organization and ritual are used in Unitas to promote interdependence. Everyone has a title which denotes the person's role in the group. Each family role carries with it responsibilities and expectations for behavior. The large family is decentralized into small symbolic families to permit an individual sense of belonging without anonymity. Decentralization spreads the source of control, with Unitas teens acting as deputies for Eismann, the "grandfather" of the extended family. It also allows for some degree of flexibility to accommodate the needs of different kinds of children and different parenting styles among the teenagers.

The drama of the extended family circle ritual, based on the symbolic family structure, is a communicative as well as an aesthetic act, functioning to reinforce values which serve to unite the group and to provide reassurance and relief of tensions prevalent in everyday life. It comprises everything from Eismann's poetic introductions and conclusions in family circle meetings, to the formation of the circle, and to the various standard directives and invocations, such as "I will know you are ready (to hear me speak) by your silence." Ritual also includes the mundane regularities of ordinary procedure, such as meeting in the same place on certain days and at certain times, and sitting with the same people.

The extended family circle convenes once each week during the school year and four times each week during the summer. The children, assisted by their symbolic relatives, arrive at the appointed hour and go to their appointed places in the Unitas circle. As soon as everyone is seated in the circle -- there may be as many as 120 children and 30 teenage and adult caretakers present -- Eismann begins the meeting. Sitting with slightly bowed head, Eismann suddenly looks up. "When you're ready I will know by your silence." The group quiets down, hushing each other, parents arranging their children in tight clusters about themselves along the circle border.

> This is Unitas. It is a program that helps children to help each other...

Although the words may vary from session to session, the meaning remains constant. Some children are creating a small disturbance which has not yet been quelled by their family members. Eismann turns his head towards them, raises his voice and points: "Did you hear me over there?" The circle is once again quiet, and Eismann continues:

> It's a program that helps children to help each other... It's like in a family where all the members help each other so that Mom doesn't have to do all the work. So that not all the work has to be done by the aunts and uncles or brothers or sisters. It's a great big family made up of little families.

He speaks easily but emphatically, enunciating clearly, as might a minister, not needing to shout to be heard by his respectful and attentive audience. Motioning with broad round arm movements, he directs his attention to each of the clusters of children and teenage parents:

> There's a family over here. And there, I see another family...Over there, there's a family...

Soon, all of the fifteen families have been distinguished.

> Unitas is made up of families to be one big family. We break bread together. A loaf of bread can be broken in pieces, but is still a loaf of bread. One big family divided in smaller families, but still one big family. Bread is for the nourishment of the body. We are here to nourish and help each other. I will now look around to make eye contact with every single person.

Eismann lifts his arm and points straight out, slowly sweeping it to single out everyone in the circle, looking intently at each person as he passes, remaining fixed on that person until eye contact is made. Occasionally, a child must be prodded and directed to look at Eismann, who is waiting, pointing at him. As Eismann does so, each child seems to emerge from the crowded circle as a distinct individual, serious and dignified. Eismann asks that those who have something to say raise their hands when eye contact is made. Perhaps ten children raise their hands. One introduces friends to the group; another complains that someone has not visited her in a long time; another explains that he must leave early today and hopes the group will understand. A staff member reminds everyone to pick up their garbage and place it in the trash cans before they leave. Much of what is brought up is mundane, apparently trivial, and some children yawn and fidget. Eismann carefully listens and responds to each word, dignifying the speaker with his individual attention.

On this particular day, Eismann has decided to lead the circle into a discussion of the family and friendship.

> As you know, the reason we have families is so that the children can be taken care of. Our mothers and fathers take care of us in the family. The reason we have families is so that the children can be taken care of.

Repetition, within one meeting and from meeting to meeting, emphasizes the important messages of Unitas, assuring that they will not be lost, and creates continuity from one session to the next.

> Who in the family takes care of us besides our mothers and fathers?

A boy from Carlos' family raises his hand and responds: "Everybody in the family." Eismann repeats, "Everybody in the family. Yes. Like who?" The boy, unsure of himself, finds safety in his first answer, "Everybody." Eismann, seeing the difficulty this child is having, but not wanting to focus on it at the moment, again repeats the response, and turns his attention to the larger circle. "So, you say that everybody helps in the family. Who else?" An eight-year-old Puerto Rican boy responds, "The aunts and uncles." Although relatively little has been said, Eismann takes this opportunity to summarize the interactions so far.

> Okay, so we have a thought going. In a family the aunts and uncles take care of us, and everybody helps out. Who else helps take care of the family?

Alina, a nine-year-old girl, bellows out, "The older brothers and sisters." A few minutes later, the grandfather is added to the list of those who help out in the family and a short discussion of the grandfather's role follows. One boy comments that the grandfather separates the children when they fight. This idea smooths a transition into a discussion of what to do when a fight begins. More children and teenagers are now eager to participate but Eismann does not allow a flowing, open discussion to develop. He seizes upon every statement, taking every word and every child seriously and deserving of full attention.

Lisa, a bashful girl in the second grade, wants to say something but seems unable to raise her voice so that she can be heard. Eismann now works to help her speak up -- no small feat for this young newcomer to Unitas, in front of over one hundred people. He does not directly encourage her himself, but asks others, first of all, her friend Maria, to help her answer through encouragement, not by answering for her. Eismann then reminds the group, "We are here to help each other, to have communication." Finally, after many attempts, Lisa manages nervously to express her thought to the group. Eismann tells the family, "She has done wonderfully. And we want to help her do it even better." Lisa has been helped to speak up publicly, praised for doing it, and encouraged to continue to work on this.

The discussion now centers on how to resolve a fight, not necessarily within a family, with children offering solutions to a hypothetical situation which Eismann describes. He has the group imagine that Nelida was very upset because someone was calling her names, and then asks the family members what they would advise her. In typical fashion, Eismann repeats what each child says, both to check that he understood and to reinforce the communication. Now and then he steps in to make a point as when Henry suggests that Nelida "call him a name back." Eismann pointedly asks, "You mean give them a taste of their own medicine? What do you think would happen if you called him a name back?" Henry thinks for a moment, then concedes, "There'd be a fight." This line of reasoning is dropped since it is obvious that retaliation will not resolve the problem.

Next, a girl suggests that the children who are fighting go to an older person to talk about their problem. To emphasize this idea, Eismann asks Terry, an experienced Unitas "parent," to repeat what the girl has just said. Paraphrasing is frequently employed in Unitas, especially if the emotional content of the utterance is high.

To emphasize the importance of friendship and communication, Eismann selects children from different Unitas families, inviting them to choose others in their families to talk to about the things on their minds. With their partners, these children come to the center of the large circle, where they are instructed to face each other to talk. With role models in front of them, everyone in the large circle is asked to do the same thing within their small family unit. Eismann then summarizes:

> Everybody needs a friend. Sometimes you can find a friend in your real family at home. That's great. Sometimes you can't. No big deal. That's okay. Sometimes you can find a friend outside of your family. Something you can do when you get angry is what was suggested over here -- you can go to a friend to talk about what happened.

Eismann pauses, looks around, and continues to make his message clear.

> To make sure that you've really understood what I've just said, can anybody say what it is that I've just said?

After a silence, Douglas, a psychodramatist who has volunteered his time at Unitas for the past year, responds: "When you're in trouble don't keep it to yourself. Take it to a friend." Eismann then asks "Who heard Douglas?" Julio repeats what Douglas said, then several other children do the same, each eager to show that he or she has understood and remembered the message.

On this positive note, Eismann announces that it is time to play. The children have about 45 minutes, until five o'clock, to play independently, not necessarily with their symbolic family members, in indoor and outdoor sports, painting and drawing, reading, board games, and blocks.

The circle reconvenes briefly at 5:15. Following a routine of many months, Eismann explicitly justifies this portion of the session to the group.

> The reason we meet at the end like this in a circle is to give any last minute messages you'd like and to have the lost-and-found. If anyone lost anything, say what it was and if anyone found anything, say what it was. I'll go around the circle and please say what

it is that you lost or found.

A pencil is reported missing, a blue jacket is found and returned to its owner who, after urging from his family, thanks the boy who found it. Sally, a symbolic mother and psychodramatist, asks one of her children on the other side of the room why she has not come to sit with her family. She suggests that Anna speak with her about it afterwards. Eismann pulls together the session in his comment to Sally.

> I like your idea that when someone has a problem they might like to talk to someone about it. It brings us back to what we were talking about. Maybe if Anna has something she'd like to talk to you about, you could get together and she could tell you about it. That brings us back to what we were talking about before.

Today is Margaret's last day at Unitas and she expresses her sadness about leaving. Once each week for two years, Margaret has been volunteering her time as an art therapist, working with children during play time. The circle applauds as they often do when someone makes an announcement of an important life change, such as a birthday. But the applause this time is half-hearted. Eismann interrupts the group's response:

> It's hard to clap when someone you know is leaving us. It's kind of hard to clap. I feel sad. Margaret has been here for two years...

Margaret readily agrees to Eismann's request that she leave her phone number and address with him so that anyone who wants to can contact her. To the group, Eismann then adds: "If you want to say anything special to Margaret you can say it to her in your own special way." Goodbyes are sad and the children are encouraged to recognize this, but they are also taught that bonds with people you love remain strong even though the people may be gone.

Once each May, at the time when the social work students complete their year of internship at Unitas and other mental health workers leave, the program conducts a "breaking of the bread" ceremony. The lessons of this ceremony, held as part of the extended family circle meeting, are the lessons of Unitas: human interdependence, the unity of life, and the strength of love. A loaf of bread becomes the symbol of the Unitas family and friendship. Each year Eismann tells a tale -- fashioned on a Biblical story (Luke 24) enacted in pantomime by the teens in the middle of the circle -- of two men on a country road, saddened by the death of their friend. Before his death, the friend would take bread, break it, and give it to the two men, saying, "Eat this bread and remember me and I will be with you." A stranger speaks with the travelers on the road, then takes a loaf of bread and shares it with them. When they look into the face of the stranger, they see that he is their friend.

> When you break bread, remember each other. The bread is not many breads, it is one loaf of bread. We are one family. But know that you can take the bread and break it into little pieces. The bread and we are alike. If we break the bread and share it with each other, then it's like having a piece of each other. Today, we break bread as a sign of friendship.

Eismann instructs the symbolic parents who are leaving to break bread with the family and remember them. The symbolic mothers and fathers are then asked to come to the center of the Unitas circle to receive loaves of bread. Eismann hands every "parent" a piece of bread, telling each of them, "Feed yourself and feed your children." But first, as the "grandfather" of the family and the "father" of the Unitas parents, he breaks off a small piece of the loaf for the "parent" to give to his "child." When all the "parents" have their loaves of bread in hand, they are instructed, for the entire extended family to hear,

> Mothers and fathers, when I give you the bread, break off chunks for the aunts, uncles, and older children. Don't break the bread for everyone. Let the aunts, uncles, and older children share the bread with the younger children.
>
> Mothers and fathers, teach your children that whenever they take bread and eat it, it is a sign of love and friendship. Go and show your children...

The children cannot contain their excitement any longer; they drown out Eismann's sentence with their eager conversation, exclamations, and pursuit of their "parents" as they return to their small family groupings.

As the extended family circle continues, children express their feelings of love and friendship toward the symbolic parents who are leaving. No negative feelings emerge during this time. Anti-social, non-group-oriented feelings are actively discouraged within the large group sessions by the lack of attention they receive. The boy who suggested that Nelida retaliate in kind against the person who called her names was pointedly discouraged from pursuing that way of thinking. Just as Unitas attempts to evaluate its participants and their behavior in the healthiest, most non-pathologic light, so, too, it seeks to cultivate the strengths within them, accentuating the positive and subordinating the negative.

In addition, Unitas teaches its children important social interactional skills. Within individual therapy or family therapy, where participants are constant and therapeutic interaction is ongoing for all, it would be appropriate to express anti-social, hostile sentiments. However, within the very large group composed of a changing cast of characters, it is inappropriate to encourage negative feelings, which is not to deny their existence. Rather, it is to suggest that they need not be foremost in highly ritual, social situations. Implicit is the idea that children suffering from a lack of external structure need to develop internalized controls, a capacity for planning and foresight, reflection upon feelings, ability to concentrate, and elementary social skills. The extended family circle provides children with a highly structured environment in which they may learn to handle interactional problems effectively, focusing on the goal of creating greater harmony, friendship, and love.

There are two ways, not mutually exclusive, to view the fact that Eismann has been the sole director of the meeting thus far. First, it might be argued that, as the main force behind Unitas, he has the training and experience to run the sessions with great facility. However, there are times when Eismann, for reasons of health or other commitments, cannot be present at a session. During these times, the reponsibility for leading the meeting falls on one of the experienced teenage "parents." Although none of them has been formally instructed in leading 130 people in a family circle, each has grown up in Unitas and learned its lessons well. This leads to the second view of Eismann's leadership of the meeting. These structured sessions and Eismann's behavior within them function as models for the teenagers in the organization of ritual therapeutic meetings. The older teenage boys emulate Eismann as the elder of the family, and it is reasonable that they aspire to be like him, to direct the sessions as he does. It comes as no surprise, then, that inner-circle teenagers speak of planning to become psychologists and social workers when they get older. Training in Unitas, just as therapy, does not take place only in formal sessions, although these are extremely important in instructing the teenagers in psychological concepts and skills.

B. *Individual Therapy*

Individual treatment sessions include psychotherapy proper and one-to-one interactions centered around activities, such as playing ball or helping a child with his homework, as vehicles through which therapeutic dialogue is conducted. This type of treatment may take place on a regularly scheduled basis, from time to time, or in times of crisis only. The place of treatment may be one of the Unitas offices at St. Athanasius, the street, or the client's home. Clients include children, families, and teenage workers. Most of the clients, especially the teenagers, are averse to the idea of being in therapy, refusing to be seen on a regular basis. From January through May of 1980 Unitas determined that an average of 41 children were seen for individual psychotherapy approximately three times every month.

Individual treatment aims to prepare the child for entrance into a therapy group. This may also be a first step toward drawing the child's biological family into treatment. Some children are unable to participate in a group modality for the following reasons:

1) They are children who enact their conflicts through bizarre or violent, gross motor behavior or vocalizations, and would be disruptive to the group. They are unable to abide by basic rules or order without which there can be no constructive group interaction.

2) The parents are non-cooperative regarding treatment either as participants in family therapy or in permitting their child to take part in a group.

3) The problem of the particular child may not be appropriate for resolution in a group context either because the nature of the child's life experience and deprivations require the closeness and intensity of a one-to-one approach, or because the problem pertains to private matters that could not benefically be shared with others, such as in the case of sexual problems.

Individual treatment provides a means for establishing firm rapport between one child and one worker. Subsequently, this bond can be used by the worker to lead the child into the family circle and the play activities, or into a small therapy group. The bond between worker and child can also be used to respond to the child individually when he provokes a crisis in the group. An example is provided by a core group member:

> One afternoon, Doc was so fed up with Bob's disrespectful behavior that, out of character and regretting it afterwards, he swatted him right in front of the family circle. Bob was infuriated with shame and seized a chair with which to hit Doc. He would have done it had not Carlos, who had formed a bond with Bob, intervened. Carlos rose, walked over to Bob and said in a low, calm voice, "Put the chair down." Bob put the chair down. Carlos often uses a strategy with Bob that Doc recommends. This is to distract him before the storm breaks by taking him

> off alone, often to get something to eat. "Hey, let's go for a pizza."

The bond that develops between a particular child and worker, regardless of whether that worker is a professional therapist or teenage symbolic parent, becomes the vehicle through which the child experiences socialization and cooperation.

C. *Play Therapy*

In a display at a local community mental health center, Eismann stated:

> In play, individually or in groups, behavior more than talk is the medium of communication. But how precious it is, for actions speak louder than words.
>
> In play, children synthesize their outer experiences; integrate internal upsets through repetitive play; sublimate libidinal and aggressive energies; enhance self-esteem through mastery; establish rules of order and norms of fair play; learn teamwork in pursuit of a goal; learn to absorb losing as well as enjoy winning; develop ever increasing levels of socialization; develop cooperation as well as autonomy; and develop a sense of initiative as they overcome a sense of helplessness.
>
> In a therapeutic setting, activities best suited to accomplish these goals are chosen. But not only is play chosen for its natural reparative function, but equally for opportunities it offers for interpretations of the meaning of behavior as it shows in the context of play interaction.

Each play therapy group at Unitas consists of 4 to 6 children, all of whom have been referred by the school they attend. The children have a range of difficulties from two or three of the broad Unitas problem categories -- acting out, withdrawn, or atypical. The groups meet once a week for one and a half hours in a local school during class hours.

The worker picks up each child from his classroom when it is time for the therapy session. The groups always meet in the same place -- in one of the school guidance suites, the nurses' office, or in an empty classroom. The end of the school year marks the termination of the groups. If a connection with the child's family has been made by that time -- an important aim -- the child may also be seen in the Unitas summer program and in meetings with the family. Some children will continue in a newly constituted group the following school year if the teacher requests it. Stekas reports that the withdrawn children generally do better in these groups than the acting-out children, as measured by teachers' ratings of their students before and after their participation in the therapy program; some children who participated showed no improvement.

The Unitas play therapy leader comes to the school with a "suitcase as a traveling clinic," according to Eismann, stocked with the materials of play therapy: drawing paper, pencils, crayons, small plastic farm and jungle animals, a toy telephone, clay, toy soldiers, a ball or two, and jacks. No board games are included since they are considered to afford only "low level therapy." They are provided only for those children for whom less structured toys are too threatening, eliciting frightening fantasies in a particular child. Such children will be seen preferably on a one-to-one basis rather than in group sessions.

The role of the worker is to connect what he knows about the child's past to the child's choice of play materials and to the content of his play. The worker will say things to the children to help them understand what they are doing and why. He will connect his observations of a particular child's play with the concerns of other children in the group, perhaps clarifying what the child is doing in terms of his or her role in the group. Thus, if the child is using a jungle animal to attack a farm animal, the worker may observe that the other children may sometimes feel like the farm animal when this child attacks them.

The worker's interpretations remain close to the child's symbolic level. Thus, the worker can clarify the child's activity by putting into words what the child is expressing through play while using the child's own metaphor. Otherwise, according to Eismann, "You will lose the kid." For example, if the worker perceives the child's play in terms of his conflict with the mother, he will refrain from saying, "Maybe that's what Mother does at home," since the child is playing with toy pigs, not a mother doll. Instead, the worker will comment to the group as a whole, "The little pigs are scared of the mother pig." Later on, when the connection with the human mother is closer to the child's conscious thought, the worker may drop the word "pig" in talking about the feared mother.

What happens if the children fight over the materials? Permissiveness does not reign. Play group therapy is not a purely cathartic experience behaviorally without limitations of any kind. A major aim is to strengthen and build the child's ego functioning, that is, to teach him to take certain realities, such as time limitations, respect for materials and other people, into account before acting. The major strategy to achieve this, reflecting the Unitas belief in interdependence, is to help the children to be helpers and controllers of each other. Eismann considers this a unique contribution to play therapy. Rather than solve the problem at hand, he urges the children to seek solutions themselves by teaching them how to deal with each other, telling them what to say and when. Eismann presents it as follows:

> Two children are fighting over the use of the jungle animals. What is to be done that will be both therapeutic and sound social conduct? The worker observes: "You both want the jungle animals. Two people want the same thing at the same time."

In the parlance of clinical interviewing, the worker is "reflecting" what is going on. A deceptively simple tool, but far removed from head-on attempts to do something about the situation, such as, "Well, wait until she is finished, then you can have your turn." Eismann continues:

> The worker then turns to the other children in the group. "What can they do about this?" If no one comes up with anything, the worker may cue the child himself: "I have an idea. You know what it is? Ask him how long he's going to play with it. He says he doesn't know? Then ask him, 'Well, when you're finished, can you let me play with it?' "

Always more important for Unitas than the immediate solution of any problem is to convey to the child and make his own the attitude that there are reasonable ways of accomplishing things through the child's own resources, to build up a repertoire of behaviors that will provide the child with flexibility and a sense of competence and self-confidence, and that will, above all, bring children together in harmonious relationships setting a pattern for their lives outside and in the future.

D. *Classroom Therapy*

Each year, Eismann runs classroom therapy groups at St. Athanasius. In 1978-79 he led two such groups. The classroom group is run along the same lines as the family circle. Eismann opens the meeting with the same ritual: "The reason we're meeting together is to talk about the concerns that sixth grade people have about lots of things." As in the family circle, he directs his attention around the classroom, pointing to each student, acknowledging those who volunteer to say something. The agenda consists of classroom and interpersonal incidents or particular students' attitudes and behaviors. Sometimes Eismann continues a discussion of a topic raised in a previous session.

One goal of the classroom therapy sessions is familiar, as stated by Eismann:

> ...let me go into that classroom where those problem kids are together with the other kids who you say are not problem kids. And let me see how I can work together with that whole class and the teacher and try to create a climate in the class so that the troubled kids can be helped not so much by me, but by what I stir up in the healthy kids to have an influence on the others.

A closely related aim, just recently undertaken, is "networking" the children, putting them in structured contact with each other, class to class, grade to grade, by establishing, for example, regular meetings between upper and lower graders. In 1980-81, 18 upper graders at St. Athanasius were linked to 36 lower graders who had a variety of academic and interpersonal problems, as perceived by their teachers. Such linkages, organized around tutoring after school, aim to create a friendship bond for these needy young children. The older "mentors" are supervised by Eismann in order to achieve the goal of this pairing arrangement, namely, to heal loneliness, shyness, or attention-getting behavior through a friendly relationship with an older person.

In the classroom group, the elementary school teacher must be present not as a co-leader with Eismann, but as a participant. Concomitant seminars with teachers alone are conducted to further their understanding of the group sessions and to provide them with ongoing supervision of their own work with pupils.

A brief description follows of a portion of a classroom therapy session conducted by Eismann with thirty children in a sixth grade class and their teacher. Toward the end of this class therapy session, Carmen finally works up enough courage to bring up something that has been bothering her very much. Others have been speaking their minds, perhaps providing Carmen with the encouragement she needed. She tells of how she had an argument yesterday with Martha in the lunchroom and accidentally broke her eight dollar record, which she now has to replace. She expresses how angry she is at Martha who always seems to have the advantage. A struggle now occurs between the two girls, each expressing her anger at the other. Eismann interrupts, saying, "You're both angry, perhaps even hurt, but screaming at each other is not helpful. Let's try another way." Eismann then asks each girl to think of two things she does not like about the way the other treats her and to say them to each other. Carmen begins by stating that Martha thinks she is best in everything, a show-off who "thinks she can get any boy in the school." Reframing what she said, Eismann comments that, while, of course, she should think well of herself, Carmen would like it more if Martha could be aware that other people also have good things to show off about themselves. To the rest of the class, Eismann notes that when people are growing up they feel proud of the way their bodies begin to look and like admiration from others. Sometimes, he adds, children worry when their bodies are not developing as quickly. It is now Martha's turn. She claims that Carmen always "acts like a baby" and "cracks her knuckles." Again Eismann reframes: "Carmen is a young lady, but there is a baby part of her that shows frequently. All of us have a baby part. It is hard growing up, wanting to and not wanting to at the same time. Does anyone know what I mean?" Several students elaborate on this, reinforcing Eismann's tactic to neutralize the anger between the two girls by surfacing their growing-up concerns about sexuality and self-image.

In closing the session, Eismann comments to the class on the courage these girls had to talk to each other in front of everyone. "They do not have to agree with each other's viewpoint, but can listen and sort out what might be useful to learn about oneself." Indeed, Martha and Carmen were given an opportunity to perceive each other as "co-travelers" struggling with issues of maturation rather than as enemies with divided agendas. Again, the goals of Unitas are reflected: cooperation, mutual helpfulness, interdependence, and focus on growth, not pathology.

E. *Art Therapy and Remedial Reading*

Art therapy and remedial reading groups have had checkered success at Unitas, partly because of poor planning, an inadequate referral system, and a lack of competent staff to run these programs. In February of 1979 Unitas handpicked a group of "most chronic youngsters" to receive a package of various therapies, including either art therapy or remedial reading four days a week for two hours after school. Each child was paired with a volunteer teenager who was receiving on-the-job training in these special treatment modalities. This program failed, according to Unitas, because

> ...choosing the most severely disturbed children to come to a structured remedial program four days per week was too high an expectation. Due to the severe performance limitations in academic, visual, coordination, and basic skills, their progress, according to our consultants, was not significant.
>
> The remedial education consultant evaluated the real gains to be in the training of our volunteer teenagers who could now duplicate part of her program themselves. The art therapist conversely judged the volunteers in her program as being themselves in need of an art experience, therefore, not ready to take leadership in the art therapy program.

For these reasons, Unitas changed the art program drastically. For the summer cycle of 1979 Unitas hired an art therapist to run the art therapy section of play time after the extended family circle. At the end of the summer, arrangements were made to develop, for Unitas' winter cycle, a new art therapy program which would be open not to a carefully chosen few, but to all Unitas children.

Each day, two or three symbolic families come to the art room to create art together, as a family. Milk and cookies, provided by the program, and in keeping with the nurturing experience of Unitas' clinical thinking, enhance the afternoon's experience. This program has been highly successful, with average attendance reported of 82 to 91 percent. If a child does not attend, his or her surrogate teen parent does outreach into their homes.

The remedial reading program did not share the fate of the art therapy program. In spite of its potential for success, the remedial reading component of Unitas was not developed with the same strong support as the art therapy program. After the initial failure, Eismann suggested that individual tutoring might be offered during school time, several hours each week, by experienced teenagers. Such a program was initiated during 1978-79 through the Urban Corps, a city agency employing low-income college students to work in one of its intern sites. Unitas teens, now in college, were able to work with their symbolic children in need of remedial help, up to 20 hours a week during school time.

In addition to this remedial education program, other teen "parents" established a second program, organized by Neil, an up-and-coming "parent." This is significant as an indicator of the increasing power of teenagers and other workers within Unitas. High attendance rates and improved reading, math, language arts, science and social studies skills attest to the success of this program, although the important gains made were in terms of the relationship of the children and the surrogate parents. According to Unitas' assessment:

The main thrust of this program was not tutoring but to expand the involvement the teenage surrogates have with the children. The goals were to afford the children individual attention from their Unitas parents, some homework help, and a half-hour play period.

F. *Family Therapy, Family Work, and Advocacy*

Family therapy sessions, when conducted, are held every week or two. The aim is to sit down with the family, identify work that needs to be done in terms of problems in the relationships among all members, and attempt to solve them by restructuring the family relationships. In order to be carried out, family therapy requires a commitment on the family's part and regular attendance at sessions.

Sessions are usually held in the family's home, rarely taking place at Unitas offices in St. Athanasius. Stekas feels that families fail to attend sessions held outside of their homes mainly because of traditional resistance to intervention and practical constraints, such as the presence of young children in the family whom mothers do not want to take out into the mid-winter cold. Families feel more encouraged to participate when the workers go to them. This sets the workers apart from the kind of contacts such families have had at a multitude of agencies, hospitals, and in the schools.

In beginning family therapy, Unitas sometimes arranges a meeting of the child's social network, which may include, in addition to his immediate family, relatives not in the home, neighbors, friends, teachers, and the school guidance counselor. The aim is to explore the human resources in the child's life. Usually, someone is discovered who has rapport with the child, who can wield influence with him, and whose participation in the treatment plan will be enlisted by Unitas.

Between December 1978 and April 1979 an average of 28 families were treated in family therapy, with an average of three or four individuals present at each session. One year later, between January and May 1980, this number had decreased to 20 families, due to a shortage of trained staff.

Many families are unable to make the commitment to the concerted, organized effort which constitutes family therapy. A number of families are headed by a mother overburdened by the concerns of little money, many children, little or no vocational preparation and a tendency to resign herself to her fate. In Unitas' terms, these families are in a state of collapse, the parents have all but resigned from their parenting functions and have sunk into profound apathy. Unitas sees such families for what it calls family work. Family work is also the natural antecedent to family therapy. There is no distinction between family work and therapy in terms of frequency or regularity. However, family work often involves contacts during times of crisis, such as when a child has been in an accident or is in trouble with the school, giving such work a frenetic, emergency-room character.

A third type of work done with families is advocacy. Unlike family work, advocacy does not explicitly aim at eventually bringing families into family therapy. Rather, a specific, short-term goal is established and work towards it begun. An example of advocacy is if a child needs to be taken to a hospital for tests but there is no one available at home to do this, or perhaps the family members available are monolingual in Spanish and an interpreter is necessary. Once the tests are completed, the advocacy role of the Unitas worker ends.

Many of the family contacts made by Unitas staff involve a combination of family work, family therapy, and advocacy. For example, Garcia, a B.A.-level social worker, visits the Rodriguez family regularly every two weeks. His family work with them has many goals, such as to help them obtain Medicaid for an adopted child, and to convince the mother that her son needs glasses. It involves some supportiveness, such as asking after family members' health and helping them out in everyday tasks. For example, if the mother is washing the dishes when a worker pays a call, the worker is encouraged to pick up a towel and start drying; or he may help her defrost the refrigerator if that is called for. Every opportunity is taken, however, to initiate a therapeutic process; that is, to instigate a shift in the family's characteristic mode of functioning.

As of the summer of 1979, Unitas staff have been seeing fifty families for either family therapy or family work. Fifteen of these are seen weekly, thirty-five are seen every two or three weeks, the majority for family work. A few more experienced teen parents do family work but may not do family therapy, which is reserved for the professional workers.

Family Therapy Case Example: The Lopez Family.

The Lopez family consists of the father, stepmother, and four children, one of whom, the youngest, is the stepmother's own. Three of the children attend school; the fourth is still too young. Unitas received complaints from the school that the children, while not behavior problems, were coming to class without notebooks and looking neglected. The most serious complaint was about Helen, in kindergarten, who was stealing money. The Lopez children had been coming to the Unitas family circle all along, where they seemed to behave well.

Sanchez and Stekas went to visit the Lopez family in their home. On their first visit they limited themselves to explaining what Unitas was all about and to talking about the children. The workers put it this way: "We are interested in children at Unitas...we visit their homes and want to get to know more about them. Sometimes when children are problems to themselves, usually the whole family feels it." The aim of this presentation was to introduce the importance of the family system, that is, the interrelationships among family members as the problem, rather than any one member.

All the children and Mrs. Lopez were at the first meeting. This gave the Unitas workers an opportunity to open the question of the upbringing of the children. The workers remarked in a pleasant, neutral way, as if taking note of the weather, "My goodness, so many children." Mrs. Lopez responded by commenting on how hard it was to handle all of them. One worker answered sympathetically, still in a non-probing, conversational vein, "I can imagine." This interchange broke the ice. Mrs. Lopez began to talk about her concerns with the children. Thus the first session followed the format of polite, social discourse with introductory expressions of good will and of benign, nonintrusive interest in comfortably shared aspects of the family's daily life.

During the second meeting, attended also by Mr. Lopez, the workers questioned the couple on the general facts of the family history. They learned that prior to the father's remarriage six months before, the children had been living apart from him and from one another in foster homes and with aunts. The father had sued for and obtained custody of the children. Now the problem seemed to center around the family's relations with the children's natural mother, who maintained sporadic contact with them. Mr. Lopez said that he was not interested in further discussing this problem with the workers and that he was taking care of this matter in his own way. Although this point was judged to be largely responsible for the children's problems, the workers' strategy was to deal directly only with the presenting problems until enough trust was established to target the central conflict.

In keeping with this strategy, at the third meeting, the workers broached the question of the teachers' complaint to the children directly: "What do you think the teachers told us about you? Tell us one good thing and one bad. Then we'll tell you what they said." Again, the workers sought a tactful way of opening a potentially antagonizing subject, while also diagnosing the children's capacity for good judgment and for realistic perception of themselves and of others. The children's answers were on target. This good fortune enabled the workers to voice the teachers' complaints while simultaneously affirming the children's positive qualities: "Helen, you know you are really right about what the teacher said." The workers attempted to make clear to the Lopez family that they were not part of the school system, nor that they necessarily shared the teachers' ideas about what the trouble was.

After several sessions, the concrete problems for which the children had been referred were practically resolved. The sibling group was encouraged to muster up self-imposed controls. Each was to see that the other fulfilled certain duties. Sanchez met weekly with the three older siblings, in the morning in an office at their school. He focused on the tasks of keeping clean and getting homework done. The children now went to school washed and with the notebooks the Unitas workers had bought for them. The workers noticed that the children, who had always participated actively in family circle meetings, two or three of them having something to say to the group each week, were asking to be heard less often. It seemed that their need for the group's attention had subsided concomitant to their participation in family therapy sessions. Helen stopped stealing after her behavior was framed in terms of an attempt to win friends by buying them candy with the stolen funds. Alternate methods of winning friends were discussed by the sibling group in an attempt to help and encourage Helen. She was offered other more acceptable means of starting a friendship.

The family had now been meeting for therapy sessions once a week for two and a half months. Up until this time only issues to do with the children's homework, cleanliness, and squabbles as they came up had been talked about. Mr. and Mrs. Lopez then indicated that they wanted to deal with concerns centering around the family's relationship with Mr. Lopez's former wife. The couple brought this issue up themselves, having arranged a meeting without the children present. This took place, as always, in the couple's living room, in the early evening. When a child strayed in, the workers would direct the parents to ask him or her to leave, as adult business was being discussed. The couple brought up their differences in approach to childrearing. She tended to yell, he to be more lenient. The only boy, Mrs. Lopez's son, was overindulged, according to Mrs. Lopez, and resented by the girls. Mr. Lopez spoke of difficulties in dealing with his former wife. He could not go against her wishes, even if this meant her taking the children away on visits at inopportune times, such as during a school week. The workers helped Mr. Lopez to determine the kind of visitation privileges he felt should be set on the mother and to stand firm on them.

Up to this point, the content of the sessions, while shifting to parental conflicts had remained tied to issues directly involving the children. Subsequently, however, the couple began to talk of more personal concerns regarding their marriage. Thus, Mrs. Lopez voiced her uncertainty about Mr. Lopez's commitment to her and her ambition to return to school in preparation for a job. This became the core issue around which the family sessions were now conducted. Family therapy was now directed toward resolving the opened up area of the dysfunctional marital relationship.

As the family continued in treatment during the year, the Unitas workers framed the issue in terms of relatively normal adjustment problems of a reconstituted family; that is, a family that has reformed and taken in new members in the process, a family which must reinforce new bonds of loyalty and reconcile the newly formed couple's mutual expectations and childrearing attitudes. The focus had shifted to the couple, in line with the theory of family functioning subscribed to by Unitas, to the effect that a dysfunctional family rests on a dysfunctional marital subsystem, and also in accordance with the Lopez's own shift in concerns.

G. *Training Modalities*

1. Teenage Circle

Together with professional staff, the main therapists in Unitas are the teenagers. Several of the "teenagers," however, are actually in their early twenties, but all entered Unitas when they were either children or teens. All the teenagers are in adult roles of "parents," "aunts," or "uncles," and as such are reponsible for the children in their respective symbolic families. They are expected to treat the children with respect, sensitivity and therapeutic awareness, and to turn to one another when a difficult situation arises. Symbolic parents are more responsible than symbolic aunts and uncles, but they are not on a different level. The teens are the catalysts for change in the children. They do this through their direct contact with the children in the extended family circle, in play, and in the outside community. In order for them to understand the nature of such work and perform well, they must participate in training sessions conducted by Eismann. Training occupies an exceptionally important place within Unitas for both paid and volunteer staff.

The training of the teenagers consists of two parts: the teenagers training each other and the teaching by Eismann of the psychological concepts and skills needed to handle children effectively. Usually, these two parts are combined so that formal training by Eismann is interwoven in one session with the more informal peer interactions. The teen circle meets twice each week during the summer, for two hours each session. All teenagers who are employed full-time attend these sessions as part of their work week, as do most staff members. The presence of trained mental health workers does not change the purpose of these meetings. They function primarily to train the teens, regardless of who is present.

It is now ten o'clock on a Tuesday morning in July of 1978. Seated in chairs in a wide circle around a classroom at St. Athanasius are 35 young people, some staff, and Eismann. The stifling heat has prompted the purchase of doughnuts and cold juice for everyone by the program -- a little sustenance to lift drooping spirits. The first item of discussion revolves around the organization of Unitas. Some dissatisfaction among the staff and workers has been voiced. Trained health workers complain that the teens do not respect their use of the room. At this time only one room is available for seeing clients and for teenagers to socialize. Eismann asks the teenagers not to use the Unitas room for socializing when workers are in the room for business. He quickly adds "but friendships are important...they are what make Unitas work." Hours are then set when the room is open to all teenagers: before the morning program, during lunch, and after the afternoon circle on the street. Workers are asked to close the door to the room when it is unavailable for socializing, thus providing another clue to the teenagers of the behavior expected of them. Eismann, who usually repeats messages to insure their communication, decides to ask instead if there are any questions. Several comments later, this discussion closes. Eismann then raises the issue of bureaucracy, noting that

> Three-quarters of the families of the area here do not respond to formalities and referrals. They respond to a person's touch. For example, your child has a bad problem and the guidance counselor says, "Your son is having great problems in school and it will be necessary for him to see a professional counselor."

Eismann speaks with great formality as he mimics a school guidance counselor. He then asks the teenagers, "What might you feel if someone said this to you?"

Raul: I'd feel like I didn't raise the kid right.

Eismann: ...that you were being yelled at.

Juan: I'd be angry.

Eismann: Juan suggests that when you meet somebody who is angry with you, you get angry with them. You then do the opposite of what is asked. Nobody likes to be blamed, criticized, made to feel no good. We get defensive. In Unitas we try to reach out in a very personal way to parents and children, to empathize, to literally touch, to reach out and touch with our words.

The teenagers are being taught methods of understanding and dealing with the children in therapeutic ways, for, he explains to them,

People helping people will do better with a body of knowledge. Although it can take place without it, it is better with it.

The techniques he uses to teach the teenagers are also the techniques which they are being taught. Eismann attempts to make the teenagers put themselves in the children's shoes, by reading the children's facial expressions, gestures, tones of voice and words, in the process he calls "decoding", to arrive at the underlying motive or purpose -- that is, rationale -- behind seemingly random, annoying, or inappropriate verbalizations or behavior. He then has them practice by casting them in the role of the child, having them repeat what the child said, and then put into words the child's decoded message. This, he argues, is a powerful healing tool. How decoding can be healing is illustrated by the following example, in which Eismann demonstrates how the teenagers can heal the children, and indeed, each other and friends, by applying his method to the actual process occurring in the teen circle itself.

Eismann: There are certain people who, when you feel down and out, say certain things and you feel better. Others you stay away from. Who needs their words! (Assenting laughter from circle). But these people may be that way because that's what's said to them. Here you begin to learn the language of feeling which is the language of healing. This is not academic experience where you take a test to pass and then forget everything you know. (Chuckles from circle).

Here I'd like to provide experience for you which you will use in life. When a person comes to talk to you, try to figure out what the person feels. Words are not that important. When a person is depressed, if you get across to him that you have an idea of what it feels like to be in his shoes, then something will happen, will help him to feel mobilized again.

(To Andrea): I said I feel lousy.

(To Barbara, in a soft voice): Gee, Barbara, you really feel washed out; you feel like getting away from it all.

(To Juan): Gee, Juan, you really feel beat, don't you?

Anybody want to try an expression?

No one responds. Eismann continues to address various people from the circle, verbalizing the feelings he reads in their bodies, but not looking for a response. He is still demonstrating a technique.

(To Howard): Gee, Howard, you really feel fed up with the world today.

Other teens laugh. It is a hot, muggy day and everyone is limp.

Any other expressions?

Again, no one responds. Eismann changes his question.

Who here feels lousy today?

Many hands are raised in response to this. Teenagers begin to speak up.

Howard: I feel tired; I don't feel like doing anything...

Eismann: Andrea, you could really buy that. Say it!

Andrea: (Consumed with anxious, embarrassed, voiceless giggles each time she makes an attempt to speak as Eismann instructed her, she shields her face with her hand).

Howard (to Andrea): I can't hear you.

In both the extended family circle and teen circle meetings, all are encouraged to express their ideas and feelings clearly. Teenagers and children alike are publicly and explicitly praised for such behavior, especially if they obviously have difficulty doing it.

Andrea is looking down now, still embarrassed by the attention she is getting and her inability to speak. Eismann decides to pursue this issue in a different way. He rises from his chair, walks over to Andrea, indicating to her that she should move her chair into the center of the circle. He does the same with Howard. Then, to the rest of the circle, he says,

Eismann: When you're depressed, you talk softly. No wonder I can't hear Andrea. When you're with somebody who is depressed, don't shout. Talk softly so they will really know you know what it feels like to be in their shoes. Andrea said it so softly that you couldn't hear it at all.

Howard (repeating what he said earlier): I feel lousy. I don't really feel like doing anything.

Andrea responds to Howard but she is no longer visibly upset, as she was just a few minutes earlier. Eismann decides to bring other teenagers into the interaction. He asks if someone else could come up and say that he understands what Howard feels. Eismann's question is greeted, again, with silence, but he relentlessly proceeds, without irritation or impatience.

He asks Howard to repeat what he said yet another time.

Howard: I feel lousy. I don't really feel like doing anything.

Eismann (stands behind Howard's chair and speaks for Howard): I feel lousy. This is really the pits. I don't know how I'll get through the day. If I had my way I'd go home. (Chuckles from circle. Howard nods vigorously, agreeing wholeheartedly with what Eismann has just said). Is there anyone who can say it?

Janet raises her hand and she is asked to join Howard and Andrea in the center of the circle.

Janet (to Howard): You're really feeling tired, aren't you?

Howard (to Janet): Yes.

Eismann calls on Jesus, who has raised his hand, but does not ask him to sit in the center.

Jesus: You feel hot?

Before Howard can answer, Eismann interrupts to comment on the question just asked, directing his response to Howard.

Eismann: Yes, but that's just on the skin. Deeper in, how do you feel? Howard, tell us more about how you feel, to give us ideas.

Howard: I just feel sleepy, like going home to take a nap and not wake up until tomorrow. (Snickers can be heard from the other teenagers).

Again, Eismann shifts the train of thought to get the teenagers more involved in this exercise. Asking about their current emotional state is not getting them very far - perhaps the day is too steamy and miserable for anyone to go beyond their discomfort. The day before, the entire group of teenagers, children and staff had gone to Bear Mountain State Park for a day away from the hot concrete of the city. Eismann asks about the trip.

Eismann (to Howard): Did anything happen yesterday that got to you?

Howard: No.

Eismann: Everything went okay?

Howard: Yes.

Eismann: Just tell us anything that happened yesterday.

Howard: A boy...he went too near the diving board where he was told not to go. He almost drowned. The lifeguard had to go in and get him out.

Eismann (to circle): How do you think Howard felt?

Now, a number of teenagers are ready to respond. They tell Eismann that they think Howard felt afraid, anxious, shocked.

Eismann: Afraid...anxious...shocked. Everyone who has a word for how Howard felt, come up, please.

People come into the circle and take turns sitting in the chair across from Howard, each offering him a word. When they are done, Eismann sits down in the chair opposite Howard, saying,

> Howard, people say if they had been in your shoes they would have felt anxious, afraid, shocked. Are these the kind of feelings you had? Do those words describe it?

Howard nods in assent. Again, Eismann institutes a change in the flow of the discussion.

Eismann (to circle): Now do the opposite, not supportive. Be as sarcastic as you can. (In mock aside): We are all good at that!

Janet (enthusiastically volunteers, leaping up to sit in the chair across from Howard): You should have let the kid drown!

Eismann (to Janet): Good!

Raul (taking his turn sitting in the chair): *You* couldn't have helped the kid if you tried! (Snickers from the circle).

Janet (once again taking a turn): The kid was told not to go to that part of the pool. You shouldn't have felt worried. You're not his mother or father.

It is not surprising that Janet is deriving so much pleasure from venting her spleen in this relatively safe, controlled setting. Throughout the summer, Unitas staff described Janet as an extremely angry young woman. She was gruff and insensitive to the children and to her fellow workers, who could be heard complaining to one another about her behavior. After the summer during which this meeting took place, Janet continued to volunteer at Unitas, eventually making the transition from symbolic aunt to symbolic mother status. With her continued participation and added responsibility, she has become more at ease with other workers and the children.

Eismann (to Janet): That's it! That captures it in a nutshell! (Eismann then sits in the chair opposite Howard.) (To Howard): Tell me, how did this make you feel? (He leans toward Howard and says in a low voice): We'll talk quietly, between us only. No one else has to hear.

Howard begins to relate the swimming pool incident in more detail to Eismann exclusively.

Eismann (to circle): You hear? He's telling me more about the kid, about what happened with the lifeguard. He feels better now.

Various teenagers, their curiosity aroused, want to know what Howard is saying to Eismann. Eismann does not respond directly, at least not in the way they want. The point he makes concerns form far more than content.

Eismann (to circle): We have to finish up now. The point I want to make is listen to the feeling a person is having and tell them...with children particularly. Do this with children. That will help them to behave better. When you really feel like cracking somebody in the face, try hard to understand what feeling he's having. I know it's hard. This is just a beginning... an appetizer.

Paul: What if a person doesn't know what he's feeling?

Eismann: Then you can say, "I think you don't know what you're feeling at this moment." There! You have already captured it!

Carlos: When I don't know what I'm feeling I start talking and then after talking and talking I can catch what I'm feeling so it's good just to let them talk.

Carlos has been in Unitas since he was 8 years old; he is now one of the inner core of teenagers. He makes his point in the same declarative manner as does Eismann, who neither comments on the youth's statement nor finds it necessary to reframe it, to make it clear to the other teenagers. In this regard, Carlos, and the other teenagers who have his stature within Unitas, are midway between the new, younger teens and the professional mental health workers.

Eismann (to circle): Once in training, I had a supervisor, so critical of me, I hated her!

Various voices are raised in mock shaming of Eismann: Oooh!

Eismann asks what that response meant.

Mary: Maybe you disliked her, not *hated* her.

Eismann: Mary brought up a very important point. (to Mary: What did you say? (Mary repeats herself) (to circle): That's an important point; trying to talk me out of my feeling. Maybe Mary is right that I didn't really hate her, only disliked her. I'm supposed to love everybody, not to hate anybody. Did you hear that before?

(Murmurs of assent from teenagers).

But you feel what you feel. But when you find somebody who can be with you in your feeling -- "You really hated her, didn't you?" -- When you hear that, then you don't have to hate her anymore. So if a kid says, "I hate you!" let him feel what he feels. He may not even be hating you. Maybe he's hating his father. But he feels what he feels. That doesn't mean you *act* on what you feel. If somebody says, "I really felt like killing the guy," it doesn't mean you say, "Go ahead and do it!"

The session ends and the teenagers go to lunch with the children in the gym downstairs.

Two days later, the teenagers meet again for a training session.

Gloria, a social worker who was not present at the earlier session, indicates that she would like to know what happened, her interest having been aroused by allusions made to Howard's feelings about a child drowning. Eismann suggests that Howard go to the center of the circle. Teenagers are first empathetic, this time giving a quick run-through of what happened, expressing their concern easily. This time Howard opens up not to Eismann but to Juan, an inner circle teenager who has been at Unitas for years. Again, it is an older, experienced teenager who replaces Eismann. Empathy is followed by sarcasm, except that now the teenagers are embarrassed to be so insensitive and unkind to their fellow worker. A quick summary by Eismann concludes this session.

2. *Staff Meetings*

The content, style of management and the ultimate goals of staff meetings are much the same as therapeutic community practice is for Unitas in general. This is not accidental. Following the therapeutic community model, Unitas attempts to unify its participants, blurring the ordinary distinctions between patients and staff members. All staff members have family roles within the Unitas extended family system and so are connected to one another and the children as symbolic kindred. Moreover, the inner circle teenagers, who participate in teenage training sessions and socialize with the other teenagers, are also staff members. More than anyone else, these teenagers link the professional mental health workers, who tend to be older and from outside the community, with the local teenagers and the children.

Issues which arise during staff meetings include the general functioning of the program, the teenagers' feelings about the program and improvements which might be made, the need to maintain accurate, up-to-date statistical records of children's attendance, the relationship of Unitas to St. Athanasius (which houses the program) and its staff.

Besides these formal staff meetings, informal meetings often take place daily -- especially between teenagers in the inner circle and Eismann. These teens are weekend guests from time to time at Eismann's summer house, visit him in his Bronx apartment, and stay late at Unitas, meeting with each other and with Eismann as friends more than as co-workers or employees. The teenagers, particularly with one another, live the Unitas philosophy in their daily activities. They play basketball in the St. Athanasius gym, go to the movies, party, and get together as friends to talk and share their lives. After years of serious participation in and devotion to Unitas, it comes as no surprise that these teenagers are able to carry the program's values and methods over into their outside lives. Indeed, this is the goal of Unitas, and of any therapeutic community.

H. *Techniques for Maintaining a Therapeutic Community*

Therapeutic interactions take place within the context of the symbolic family structure, within ritual parameters in the extended family circle, and in the various therapy modalities described above. The therapeutic techniques used are similar in all modalities, thus providing consistency, although individual and small group therapies offer more of a sense of intimacy than is possible from the therapeutic community at large. The following principles elaborate the basic therapeutic underpinnings of all interventions practiced in Unitas.

Principle One: Structure, order and basic anti-therapeutic prohibitions are essential to healing. Rules of conduct and discipline set the stage for therapeutic interactions. Unitas provides its children and teens with clearcut rules by which they can define the limits of what they can and cannot do as part of the program, thereby defining their own position and wants in distinction to those of the group and requiring them to exercise self-control. Role-modeling has a place here, since children internalize the standards of behavior of their models, older youths and adults, with whom they have formed an attachment. The list of prohibitions is lengthy, and is directed primarily at the teenagers who are expected to teach the policies and principles to the children. At the outset of the summer, Eismann informs the new youth workers of the basic rules:

> Now for some ground rules. Kids will do as you do. So there are ground rules -- for health reasons only -- not open to discussion:
>
> *No* drugs. Drugs are not good. It's a health point of view, a philosophy.
>
> *No* alcohol. If, in your family, it's a custom, that's fine. A little wine in your belly, as Scripture says, is fine. The saying can be misused. If the parents see one of you drinking with the kids, that's the end

of Unitas for you. It's generally agreed it's not good for kids. Maybe it's not good for adults either, but we'll leave this.

There's an accumulation of evidence throughout the world that smoking is bad for your health. Save it for when you're at home if you need to. Not even at time-out here.

Rule Number Three: Please *no* smoking.

Rule Number Four: *No* radios. When radios are permitted, people connect with the machines. It takes people away from the opportunity to communicate directly with each other. On the street, if a kid brings a radio, politely tell him to take it home. If he wants to listen, tell him to take it down the street and listen. When he doesn't need to listen anymore, he can come back...There's a time and place for it.

Rule Number Five: We're in the group to be helpers and healers for each other. When we're out there, we're helpers and healers for the *children*...to support each other, yes, but I don't want to see workers just playing with each other. Similarly, teenage workers are expected to maintain their focus on the children, not to get involved in activities for their own sake. If you're scratching someone's back and look elsewhere, talking but not looking at the person, you are out of focus.

Juan, one of the Unitas old-timer fathers, adds this rule: "No fighting...No insults." Eismann confirms him, "Yes, no physical or verbal abuse, no calling names as a way to handle a child. That's not healing."

Principle Two: All communications in Unitas aim at healing brokenness and reinforcing strengths. A number of techniques are used to achieve these goals:

a) Rules of speaking. In the case of group modalities of therapy, one person is to speak at a time, and interruptions are not permitted. If the flow of communication does not go smoothly, the children are expected to deal with whatever problem has arisen to rectify matters. Within the confines of these rules, Unitas encourages its participants to speak for themselves, articulate their feelings, and create bonds of friendship and love with others.

b) Empathy. At the base of many of the techniques of therapeutic communication used by Unitas workers is the need to empathize. Empathy involves paying attention to and acknowledging the humanity of another person, responding accurately to his or her communications. It is a means to achieve human interdependence and love. Through empathy the Unitas worker may create an intimate bond with other people.

c) Reframing. This is the reshaping of an utterance, situation, or event in order to view it in a positive vein. When, for example, the girl described in a classroom therapy session complained bitterly about another girl, Eismann repeated her words but changed the emphasis, adding a new and not inconsistent positive note to what she was saying. Reframing is related to the Unitas value of seeing the positive or healthy in the individual or situation rather than the negative or pathological.

d) Repetition. Just as ritual refers, by definition, to standardized verbalizations and behaviors, so standardization implies repetition. In Unitas, examples abound of Eismann's use of standard procedures to influence children. At every meeting, one hears "I will know you are ready by your silence," "Unitas is one big family made up of many small families," "Help each other," or slight variations on these refrains. Another kind of repetition involves Eismann drilling the children to help them to remember a special event or a change that is to occur. For example, when the summer program begins, Unitas meets at a different time. After informing the family circle as a whole, he addresses himself to one side of the circle, "When are we meeting? At what time? Where?" The children on each side of the circle repeat the answers in unison, directing their responses to those on the other side. Eismann repeats the process several times. This may seem to be no different from teaching by rote, yet it is also a ritualized group interaction, like a dance. And, like a dance performed harmoniously with synchronized steps, it instills participating performers and spectators alike with an exciting, magical feeling of oneness with others. Repetition also serves to clarify and emphasize points made during circle meetings and other therapeutic interactions, as well as insuring participation.

e) Decoding. This is another method for understanding and communicating what the other person is feeling. As a communication skill it is related to reframing and reflecting. In decoding, the therapist changes the message around to make the child know that the therapist understands what he is saying.

f) Storytelling. Eismann makes ample use of vivid anecdotes to get across points to the children in the extended family. It is general Unitas policy that children who strive to attract attention to themselves by means of distracting others during a family circle meeting or while they are busy at work or play be ignored until they participate cooperatively. However, children who are disruptively interfering rather than merely distracting the group, by picking a fight or throwing a tantrum -- perhaps about to injure themselves or others -- are given intense attention during the crisis, often by more than one Unitas parent or staff member.

The following story, told by Eismann to the assembled extended family, is particularly relevant to the children who distract and disrupt the group.

> Once upon a time on Fox Street, when the houses were still lived in, not burned out, there was a fire truck. It had a special ladder that they put up. After they put up the first ladder, they put another one on top of that and then a third extension. And when I got there they had put it up to the top of the church. You know the church? How many know the church I am referring to? (A show of hands). And there were people looking. A little boy was on top of the church I'm talking about.
>
> The little boy had jumped from the roof of the house onto the church roof and he couldn't get off. When I got there the boy was beginning to get onto the ladder. It was kind of high -- three stories. And the boy proceeded to climb down the ladder. As he came down there were cheers and claps. When he came down, the firemen came to shake his hand. The boy changed, his whole color changed. He was beaming and felt happy. And then everyone went home and that boy learned a lesson. What lesson did he learn?

The children discuss how the boy learned the wrong lesson, namely, that he could get an enormous amount of attention by climbing the rooftops. Eismann tells how the boy repeated what he had learned, until finally he was placed in a special home for children. There he learned to develop his artistic ability, became a painter, and now receives attention from people who admire his work.

Principle Three: All healing interventions aim at encouraging an individual to believe in himself and his capacities. The techniques Unitas employs regularly seek to empower the child, not the authority, with the ability and the responsibility of handling what is redefined, reflected, reframed, as his and the other child's own affair, establishing direct lines of remedial communication between them. This breaks the vicious circle of complaining to one's superior and of introducing a third party as judge or ally for self-vindication or attention-getting. This form of problem-resolution is not consistently carried out at Unitas. Eismann remains a very powerful figure, rarely challenged directly, and is the self-appointed, ultimate arbiter. He avowedly abstains from wielding his power in the form of direct intervention, however, and reserves making use of commands for times of chaos when, for example, anxiety and hyperactivity become contagious among the children. At such times, he will dictate orders or angrily voice his own personal irritation. Generally, he strives to maintain a consultancy role toward the teen parents who are expected to empower their own children directly, as Eismann aims to empower them. Yet, in setting up interactions among Unitas members, even while discouraging them from addressing themselves to each other through him, Eismann, like a stage director, is an enormously powerful center of influence.

Principle Four: Interactional conflicts are best resolved directly by the subjects themselves through activation of the interpersonal system. This refers to the opening up of communication between the people involved in an interaction. This may be done in a number of ways, such as bringing two or more of the participants into physical proximity, for example, in the center of a teen or classroom circle.

Principle Five: Parenting experiences through physical nurturance are needed by all children, particularly those in need of corrective parenting experiences. Unitas emphasizes the physical expressions of affection and caring: holding, touching, stroking, and eye contact. Feeding is also included. Symbolic parents are encouraged to give their "children" food, to nourish them physically. An important part of Unitas during the summer is lunchtime, when the teenagers sit with their "families" and share food with their "children." Teenagers' birthdays are celebrated with cakes; doughnuts and juice often accompany a training session. The teenagers learn, by example, that the offering and sharing of food can create a strong bond between people. The annual "breaking of the bread" ceremony epitomizes this belief.

Principle Six: Positive behavior is reinforced through positive response. This requires the therapist to focus interaction on a person's strengths, building on them rather than on weaknesses. It is the outlook that describes the jar as half full rather than half empty. It is often used in the family circle to encourage children to express themselves verbally before the group, to congratulate them for whatever they have managed to accomplish no matter how meager, and to affirm faith in their capacity for improvement. This bolsters their self-confidence and rewards their assertiveness by enhancing their self-image. Positive response works to undo the apathy, hostility, and self-defeatism of children for whom family and teachers tend to reserve a pessimistic view. It helps to reverse the vicious circle of failure and low self-esteem, particularly common among disadvantaged groups.

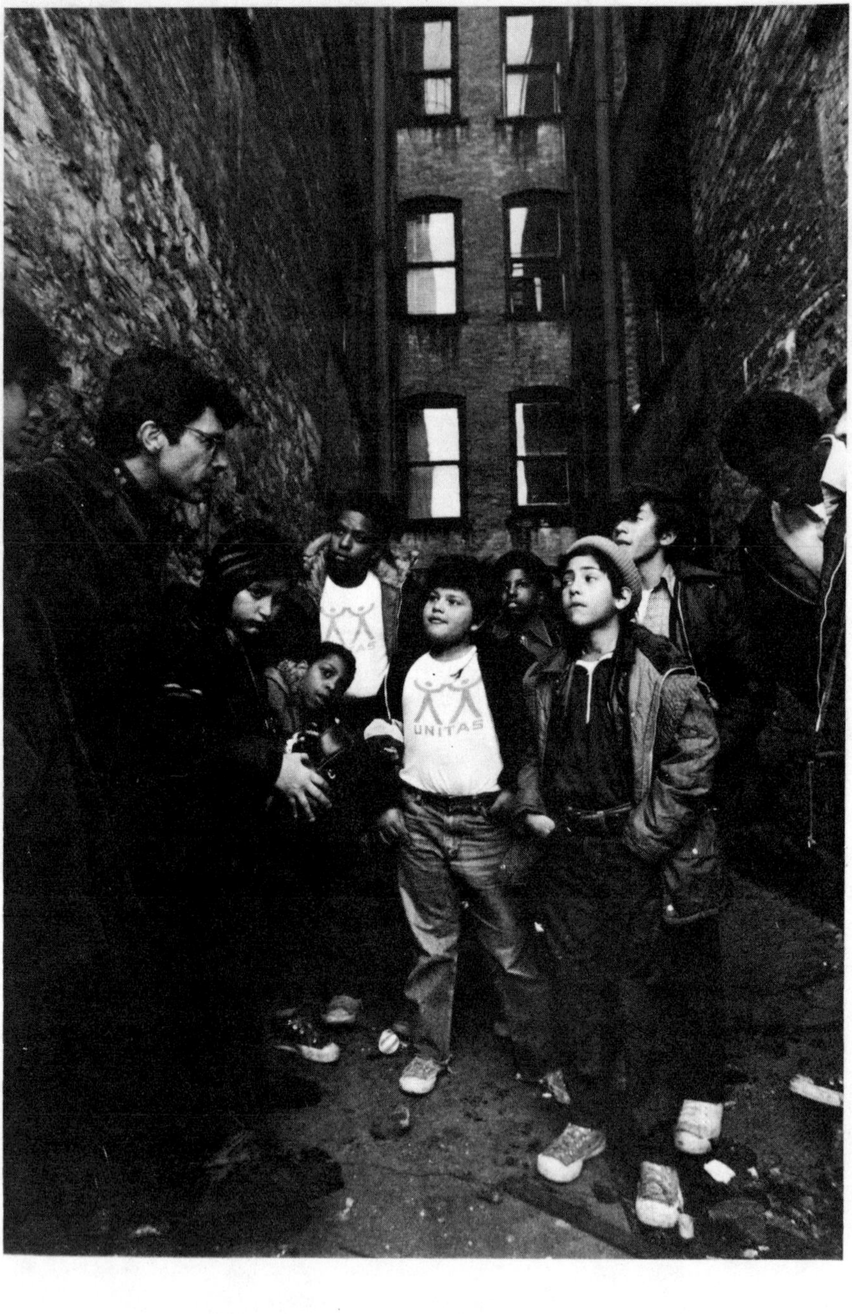

PLATE 5. Eismann attempted to bring the necessary psychotherapeutic services directly to the children in need and within the social context of that need.

IV

HISTORY OF UNITAS

The roots of Unitas can be traced back to both the history of the Community Mental Health Center movement of the 1960's and the personal development of Edward Eismann, Unitas' founder. It is at the point at which Eismann begins to develop a program based on the community mental health concept that we can best understand the shaping of the Unitas program.

What was called the "community mental health revolution"[16] of the 1960's stressed agency accountability for service utilization in a particular catchment area and encouraged the development of human resources among the client population, rather than relying solely on outside professional expertise. Animated by this innovative thrust in helping people, Eismann accepted a position at a Bronx community mental health center as a consultant in the consultation and education division. The time was January 1968 and Eismann was then 35 years old and had recently completed a clinical doctorate in social work.

During the first six months of his tenure, Eismann sat in an inadequate office in a hospital building located away from the mental health center. By Eismann's description, there was no room for anyone to sit, the hallways often doubling as office space. He passed six of his eight months at the center "waiting for something to happen." He did help to conduct four mini-workshops that were successful, but this was not enough to satisfy him. The lack of contact with community people -- he received two phone calls during his eight months at the center and saw only a handful of clients -- particularly depressed him.

Six months after he began this work, Eismann decided to go out to the street, to stop waiting for clients to come to him for consultation.

[16] Bauman, Gerald and Ruth Grunes. *Psychiatric Rehabilitation in the Ghetto.* Lexington, Mass.: D.C. Heath and Co., 1974.

> On the streets, I saw a lot of things happening. My depression began to lift. A little boy asked me, "Will you be here forever?" And from that time I saw what I was to do.

"Yes," was Eismann's reply, he would be there forever. During the summer of 1968 Eismann spent most of his time on the streets of the South Bronx getting to know the children of the area. With him was a center art therapist, also dissatisfied with being tied to the office. They selected Fox Street in the center's catchment area as a good place to begin their new work. The following is an excerpt from Eismann's notes from August 1968, when he was working with teenagers on Fox Street. The interactions of the boys with each other and with Eismann, over a two-day period, underscore the need to work continuously and closely with children on their own "turf."

August 29, 1968:

> Today the boys were playing tag. I told them to continue their game. I was happy just watching them. At a certain point they started hurling rocks and stones. I could not see their enemy, but they said it was the "niggers" from the other end of the street who had begun bothering them. I was caught in the middle of a rock-throwing party, quite anxious, and trying desperately to think of ways to distract, redirect them, or reason with them, or something. I tried thoughts with them like, "I think you have shown them enough now that they can't push you around." No reasoning helped. The war continued. Finally, it was over (I still had not seen the enemy whom the boys were saying was hiding in a certain back yard). "We won!" was the battle cry.
>
> Eddy came onto the scene and was particularly hostile, grabbing things from the boys and the boys not really defending themselves or each other against him. Eddy wanted me to see how scared he could make Howard. I expressed no interest, but he proceeded, making Howard run into his house and not emerge thereafter. It was a disheartening day in all.

August 30, 1968:

> Today I returned to the group, but found a cool reception. I was not hailed nor related to except by forced "hi's." I tried forcing conversation but to no avail. The boys who were outside were not really

> playing with each other; other boys were inside looking out the window. I knew this unsettlement between them and me, and even between them and each other, had something to do with yesterday's war. I kept hanging around, sitting on the stoop, not letting them reject me although I was feeling it. A block party was scheduled for the evening. I stayed around to be at it. When I got food, I deliberately went to several of the boys and offered them some of my food. They began coming near me again and cautiously conversing. One boy ventured to ask, "Would you beat up a kid?" I said, "Me! Why would I want to do that, I might not like what a kid does, but beat him, never." As the evening went on and I sat on the curb, four of the boys came over and "dined" with me. At last it came out. Jack said: "We thought you were real mad at us yesterday because we were throwing rocks; we thought you did not like us anymore and were not coming back." I commented that that was the way he felt, like I was through with them. Did the others feel this way too? They agreed and talked more about people who get mad at them and then are their enemies. I said, "I sure was glad you brought this up, that you were able to say these things to me." I was so pleased that they could tell me what was on their minds and how they felt. I then expressed that I was not mad at them yesterday, but I was feeling something when the rock throwing was going on. I felt afraid, not angry. Afraid that someone might get hurt and I did not want anyone of them to get hurt because I liked them. They were right, I was feeling something but it was not what they thought. It pleased me so much that we could sit here and get to understand each other better.
>
> We went over to the stoop and talked for another hour. The thoughts and feelings that emerged now were of a tender variety epitomized by Gregory who commented at a certain point: "Wouldn't it be great if we could all live together in one big house?" I said it was a beautiful thought, but at least we could be real close friends who care about each other.

Through the experiences of that summer Eismann gained a clearer understanding of what could be done to reach community members therapeutically. He requested a transfer to the outpatient unit of the mental health center where he wanted to design a children's program. However, soon after he was hired as a child clinician, the budget for the children's psychiatric services was cut, leaving no funds for the development of the new program. Undaunted, Eismann still hoped to develop a children's clientele, either by advertising with circulars or by meeting children through street contact.

There was an elementary school near the outpatient clinic but because of the lack of previous contacts there, the clinic director prohibited Eismann from approaching the administrators, teachers, or children. As he related the details of this period, Eismann's growing frustration with the priorities and constraints of the community mental health center became apparent. His overriding concerns continued to be the people of the community, especially the children, and how to reach them. He had little patience with what he perceived as the misdirected priorities of the community mental health bureaucracy.

By the spring of 1969, Eismann was known at the local junior high school, where he had been permitted to speak with people because of contacts that others had made previously. The guidance counselor referred a troubled Puerto Rican boy, Alejandro, to Eismann because of his truant behavior. Through Alejandro, Eismann met a number of other teenage boys. Eventually, Eismann's network expanded to include the boys' parents and the teachers in the school. Eismann points out that this expansion could not have occurred in such a natural easy way had he remained sitting in a clinic office waiting for clients to arrange and show up for appointments.

Also at this time, the first group of five neighborhood teenagers met with Eismann on the street. It was not long after this that Eismann chose the name Unitas for the program which he was developing with South Bronx youth. The name Unitas derives from Biblical Psalm 133 which says, *"How good and noble it is for brothers to live together in unity."* To Eismann, "mental health difficulties involve broken, unresolved relationships," and such "divided relationships are signs of divided minds. If people's heads are together, then you can be a community." Unity, thus, is projected as the goal for humans in their personal lives and their relationships with others.

Eismann held daily group and individual sessions with these boys during that summer, but they spent virtually no time in the outpatient clinic office. Meetings occurred on tenement stoops, fire escapes, at the local candy store, in the schoolyard -- wherever and whenever it made sense to talk according to the needs of the boys and not the needs of the clinic. Usually they would meet on the boys' own grounds, in the vicinity of the junior high school. With little success, Eismann tried to interest Alejandro and his friends in joining the street program on Fox Street. Although Fox Street was just a few blocks away from Alejandro's home, the children thought of it as a separate world. It was not yet time to consolidate the newly emerging program.

By this time the outreach program Eismann was developing had won the recognition and approval of his colleagues at the community mental health center. In the fall of 1969 Eismann was invited to become the acting director of children's services and to coordinate all children's activities for the center. From clinician Eismann became administrator, dealing with fifty people, most of whom were community mental health workers. Eismann accepted the position because he believed that he could build a centralized children's service where referrals could be handled effectively, a belief which was soon proven false.

His new duties curtailed his working directly with children, so Eismann transferred his cases such as Alejandro and others from Fox Street and the junior high school to clinic workers. But the workers were generally not competent, according to Eismann. They were late, often absent, antagonistic, stole from the clinic, and lacked the training and commitment to work effectively with children. Eismann found his new position frustrating since he was unable to build the kind of program he had intended and, therefore, was not displeased when his directorship ended.

In February 1970, after less than half a year as administrator, Eismann returned to being a "simple clinician" with a clear sense of relief. He soon picked up where he had left off six months earlier in his work on the streets, following up contacts and making inroads initiated at community agencies. He speaks of how he now felt free to take his "ideas from the street and bring them into buildings." The community leaders and workers whom he approached at schools, a settlement house, and a recreational center welcomed him enthusiastically. Before long, Eismann was developing various pilot programs within these institutions aimed at both staff and children using the service. In each of these projects Eismann attempted to bring the necessary psychotherapeutic services directly to the children in need and within the social context of that need. He sought to train teachers, administrators, and counselors in how to handle effectively problems of the children without automatically referring the child and his or her problem to an outside professional.

At the local elementary school, Eismann initiated a classroom therapy program in which he met with a class of children and their teachers once each week. Other teachers from the school were invited to observe but not to participate in the sessions. After each session the teachers met with Eismann in a different room to discuss what had happened during the session. At the junior high school he established a similar program in which he worked with the guidance counselor and the children in classrooms. Several months later, Eismann developed teacher-training workshops in which a dozen or so teachers met every two weeks to discuss the management of the troubled child in the classroom.

He also set up the Crisis Drop-In Center at the elementary school conceived as:

> ...a pilot program for intervening in the lives of children in the context of their own community -- the school. Children experiencing crises in the classroom can leave immediately to come to the Crisis Drop-In Center and talk and/or play out the problem which has just occurred. The child is then returned to the classroom and further efforts are made to ease the class situation which triggered the child's crisis, even by involvement of the whole class, where necessary, in discussion about why a particular child became so upset as to come to the Crisis Center.

This center, which operated two days a week, was not successful according to Eismann, for two reasons. First, the two or three community mental health workers in charge of the program were not effective as therapists. The problem of staff incompetency is one to which Eismann often refers. In this particular case the problem lay predominantly in the lack of training of the workers. They were community members selected to be mental health workers who did not have the skills necessary to understand or treat psychologically the children's problems. Faced with tasks that they were ill-prepared to handle effectively, the workers were often absent, or became anxious when faced with difficult situations. In the Crisis Center, for example, they would tend to play with the children for lack of other solutions.

The second problem with the Crisis Drop-In Center was that the teachers would send the children there simply to get them out of the classroom. The center was used not so much to help the children and the class but to punish the offending children. In retrospect, Eismann believes that "the idea was good but it wasn't thought out well enough."

There was another problem that Eismann encountered when he began to work with the children's parents: they often resisted the efforts of the community mental health workers. Parents saw them more as neighbors and peers than as professionals with the expertise to help them. Parents wanted to have their child seen by the doctor and not by just a community member. Gradually, Eismann began to rely less on the community mental health workers and more on his own direct efforts with children, community leaders, and trained professionals working in the area with children.

By 1971, Eismann had established an effective community network which could be activated to help children in need of therapeutic intervention. He tells the story of Juan Ruiz, a psychotic boy of 12 who Eismann and others sustained in the community for four years, until he was 16. Eismann worked in the school with Juan's class, with the guidance counselor, with Juan's family, and the local settlement house, where Juan went after school. During the summer, Juan participated in the Unitas Fox Street program and was watched out for by the teenagers, under Eismann's supervision. When Juan was 16, his family moved out of the neighborhood and, soon after, Juan was admitted to a state psychiatric hospital.

In the settlement house, Eismann, during the winter months, met with children from the community and from his caseload at the community mental health center, twice each week. Around a large room Eismann and his staff set up games and activities in a structured way. The staff for these activities consisted of one Neighborhood Youth Corps worker and four teenage volunteers, all of whom worked under Eismann's supervision. During the course of an afternoon, Eismann would visit each activity group. The materials used came from several sources: the settlement house, the center's petty cash fund, and the resourcefulness of the children and Eismann. Eismann has always believed that it is not the things themselves that are of significance but the interactions that take place around the materials, whether in the process of figuring out how to obtain them or in learning how to use and maintain them.

It is not difficult to see how the various components of the Unitas program as it is now structured had their precursors in the teacher's workshops, the classroom therapy sessions, and the recreational-therapeutic atmosphere of the settlement house. The catalyst, however, was Eismann's dissatisfaction with clinic work or lack of clinic work at the community mental health center coupled with an uninvolved, uncaring staff of poorly trained mental health workers.

During the early years of the Unitas program, Eismann was mainly a mediator, a direct agent who handled interactional problems between children. He soon realized that teenagers could help and perhaps be paid to do this work. In the summer of 1972, four teenage boys who had been volunteering their services received Youth Corps money to work at Unitas. Other teens continued to volunteer their time and efforts and, in subsequent years, they too were offered summer jobs in the full-time program. An added incentive for these teens, all of whom worked on a voluntary basis from September through June, was the recreational activities Eismann made sure to provide. At the mental health center, Eismann set up an unused room in a basement as a wood workshop. Teens were also given time for their own social get-togethers, to talk or play, after the day's program for the children ended. Eismann, thus, appealed to the teens on several levels -- the social, recreational, economic, and psychological -- in enlisting them into Unitas.

One of Eismann's original ideas had been to build a group home for the youngsters on the street, to keep them from being sent away to foster homes or institutions. He thought that if the very troubled children could be helped within their own neighborhood they would have a better chance of working out their problems. After pricing several houses, Eismann decided to buy a modest wood-framed house near a lake in upstate New York, about a one-hour drive from the South Bronx. Eismann then began to invite the most troubled teenagers to spend weekends there. This, however, was a short-lived project. After a week of handling psychiatrically troubled youngsters, he was obliged to spend the weekend teaching them to close the refrigerator door when they were through with it, flush the toilet, and clear the dishes from the table. He quickly decided to use trips to the lake house not as treatment for the most troubled but as a reward for the healthiest. These were the teenagers from the neighborhood who had been volunteering their time to work with children during the summers on the streets and in the winters in the settlement house. At the time of this writing, these weekend trips to Eismann's country house continue.

In 1973, Eismann became increasingly involved in the local schools, conducting more workshops with teachers and meeting with groups of children. He continued to meet regularly with teenagers at the mental health center and run the twice-weekly afternoon sessions at the settlement house. In addition, for a period of several months, he met with a group of local elementary school teachers, guidance personnel, and parents because of conflict over the parents' desire to be involved in the running of the school. Eismann describes how, by the time these weekly sessions ended, the antagonism had disappeared. His schedule also included weekly meetings with the staff at the settlement house. Meanwhile, the number of teenagers volunteering to work in the summer phase of Unitas was increasing.

In July and August 1973, in addition to running the regular street program on Fox Street, Eismann offered a 15-week seminar workshop on working with disturbed children at the local parochial school and the community mental health center. The participants, all of whom were working daily with troubled youth, included teachers from the school, workers from the Bureau of Child Welfare and the mental health center. Response to this workshop was overwhelmingly positive and led to an invitation to Eismann to work with children and teachers at the school in the fall. For a full school year Eismann ran a workshop training teachers to be therapeutic agents in their own classrooms, without referring children to outside mental health "experts." He also devised a workshop for teachers in the use of empathic communication in play therapy. This association with the parochial school continued the following year, 1974-1975.

Meanwhile, Eismann was treating children at the community mental health center but less frequently than before. More and more of his time was spent with workers and children at the settlement house and the local schools. His interests were turning away from the one-to-one therapy in which he had been trained toward working with larger numbers of people. Eismann proposed to establish a therapeutic community in the very place where people lived and not in an institutional setting. He decided to implement this plan in the spring of 1974 by inviting all the groups of children and teenagers with whom he had been working to a meeting on Fox Street. About 25 youngsters came to this first meeting at which Eismann was assisted by teenagers whom he had asked for help. At first, Eismann had doubts that this plan would work, describing it as "a crazy idea." But by this time the decision to create a therapeutic community with the still disparate groups of children was firmly made and there was no turning back.

The children were responsive and soon the Fox Street program, meeting once every week, was a reality. By the summer, Eismann had arranged to have the street closed off to traffic, creating more space for play and meetings. The youngsters went along with this, according to Eismann:

> ...because of their bondedness with me, because of their valuing my relationship to them. I was a good father and they had common identification with me.

He saw his job at this time "to help them become bonded with each other." It was during that summer that teenagers began to be called mothers and fathers rather than counselors or big brothers and sisters, as was the case until then.

Eismann believed that Unitas could be an open system on Thursday afternoons; that is, any teenagers could come provided that they took care of the younger children. The reward for doing this would be free recreation time for the teens afterwards. This new system was initiated and resulted in chaos, the teens taking over and not fulfilling their responsibilities toward the children. In order to rectify this unmanageable system, Eismann required that the teens meet for three weeks on a different day of the week, in addition to the Thursday session, for training and as a way to test their commitment. The original group of nearly 40 teenagers was soon reduced to 12.

While Unitas as an outreach program was now moving ahead successfully, the community mental health center began to experience difficulties. In 1975, with less money available for innovative work, the center's administration ordered that all outreach programs be stopped. Even before this policy declaration, however, restraints had been placed on Eismann. He was, for example, ordered to stay at the clinic more, his private office space in the basement -- and with it the workshop space that he had created for the teenagers -- was sealed. Eismann conducted a small statistical study to determine the effectiveness of the clinic in treating children of the area. From April 1976 to October 1976, Eismann found that the mean intake in one of the center's three outpatient units was scandalously low, with only 1.8 children per month seen per worker. He writes:

> It seems incredible that the catchment area with the largest children's population and the most serious needs, according to a study made by the Albert Einstein College of Medicine in 1974-75, should be so untouched by its essential source of community psychiatric help. It seems obvious that the approach of having youth come into a psychiatric facility is neither popular nor serviceable in terms of what they need.

This finding, coupled with the recent mandate that outreach programs cease, reinforced Eismann's growing conviction that he must move to make the Unitas program independent of the community mental health center. Furthermore, federal funding for the mental health center ceased in June 1976 and the center became primarily a Medicaid clinic, no longer able to sponsor Unitas.

The Unitas program continued on a part-time basis while Eismann took the necessary steps to create an organization that would function independently. A Board of Directors was organized, consisting primarily of South Bronx community leaders who had been involved in Unitas and older Unitas participants. Unitas became incorporated with the Board of Social Welfare as a charitable organization and proceeded to apply to various foundations and corporations for financial support to begin in the spring of 1977. The Greater New York Fund (GNYF) and the New York Community Trust Fund (NYCTF) approved Unitas' request for financial support, amounting to $55,000, and Chemical Bank provided additional support in donations of $2,000 and office equipment.

Eismann severed all ties with the mental health center at the end of June 1977. He was finally free to work full-time on Unitas, now officially the "Unitas Therapeutic Community, Inc.," organizationally and financially independent of major institutional restraints.

It was primarily its outreach thrust that enabled the Unitas program to get off to a healthy start. We cannot, however, discount the nine years that Eismann had already dedicated to building the program and sharing the fruits of his labor with others involved in community service. He had, by this time, a small but dedicated following of teenagers and children who helped recruit others into the program.

Unitas also owes much to other community organizations which helped it survive during these early times of independence, foremost among them, St. Athanasius and Casita Maria Settlement House. For several years, Eismann had been in close contact with teachers and administrators at St. Athanasius, where he ran workshops, worked with problem children and their families, did and taught play therapy. Unitas began to use the school gym in 1975 for its Thursday afternoon extended family circle meetings. Then, in September 1977, Eismann was granted permission to use the school's offices and classrooms on a regular, daily basis as Unitas headquarters. For nearly one and a half years, while funds were extremely tight, Unitas paid no rent for the use of this space.

With available budget funds of 1977-78, Eismann hired a full-time MSW social worker who specialized in family therapy. A teenager who began participating in Unitas in 1976 was offered a salary as a Unitas Youth Corps worker, a position which he held for six months. After this period, another youth took over the Youth Corps position for three months. With the exception of government monies available to pay teenagers during the summer, e.g., Youth Employment Program positions, and the salaries paid to Eismann and the MSW social worker, there were no paid staff members at Unitas during its first year of independent operation.

Funding has proven to be one of Unitas' greatest problems thus far, and any study of the agency's functioning must include a discussion of its financial history. As funding for the first year was drawing to an end, Eismann, basically and by preference a clinician, found himself in the position of having to search for funds to insure Unitas' existence as a functioning agency. At first unsuccessful in his attempts to get Unitas refunded, he did secure permission from the New York Community Trust to use monies left over from the grant they had given to support the program during the coming summer. These funds, amounting to several thousand dollars, were supplemented by consultation fees which Eismann was receiving for services he provided weekly at a family counseling agency. This combination of funds enabled Unitas to continue functioning throughout July and August of 1978 with its staff and program intact.

Unitas had applied to the Greater New York Fund (GNYF) and

the New York Community Trust for continued financial support from July 1978 to June 1979, but the GNYF, displeased with the fiscal management of Unitas, in which Eismann was no expert, required that an administrator be hired if refunding was to be forthcoming. In addition, Eismann learned late in the spring of 1978 -- as Unitas' funding was ending -- that the New York State Division for Youth, in conjuction with the New York City Youth Board, would be willing to match any funds that Unitas could secure. It was not until the middle of the summer that the details of this matching program were clearly known to Unitas. By this time, however, it was too late to apply for funds for the fiscal year beginning in June 1978. The four agencies involved in possible funding were on different fiscal timetables, further complicating matters.

September found Unitas without money for staff, programming, or supplies, a situation which prevailed for four months through December 1978. To cope with this, the agency eliminated all but the most basic aspects of the program. All salaries were stopped. Eismann began to collect unemployment insurance but continued working as a consultant for the family counseling agency. As he had done in the past, he directed the fees from these weekly consultations into Unitas. A B.A.-level social worker, Garcia, worked with the understanding that he would be paid as soon as there was money available. During this period, however, in emergencies Eismann paid Garcia from his own pocket. A number of dedicated teenagers continued to work at Unitas, doing whatever clerical, physical, and therapy work was demanded to keep the program functioning. Only one teenager, who had been in Unitas for five years, received federal CETA funds. In addition, two MSW students from New York University interned at Unitas from September 1978 until May 1979. Their work, for which they received no salaries, included running small therapy groups and seeing individuals and families in treatment.

The Thursday circle was maintained, as was outreach work with individuals, families, and local schools. Special programs such as art therapy and remedial reading, both of which required consultants' fees and materials, were temporarily cut out. No money was spent on rent or supplies. St. Athanasius contributed space and overhead and the program survived on whatever supplies remained from its more lucrative days.

During this period, Eismann secured funds from the GNYF, the NYCT, and matching grants from the New York State Division for Youth, through the New York City Youth Board. The total Unitas budget for the period January to December of 1979 was $85,039. Working staff began to be paid and Eismann recruited a full-time administrator (who was also a trained psychotherapist) in keeping with the agency's needs and the GNYF's requirements. In all, for the three-year period of June 1977 through June 1980, the GNYF gave grants to Unitas totalling $55,000, with the amount of the grant reduced considerably each year.

Ironically, the features which make Unitas' approach to community therapy unique have worked against its chances of being funded. The agency has proven its viability and, through its popularity and from various evaluation measures, its success. Unitas has not, however, been willing to modify its programs to allow it to fit into the traditionally oriented mental health establishment. It has, for example, turned down an offer to be affiliated with a community mental health clinic, which would make it eligible to receive Medicaid funds. Such proposals hold little appeal for Eismann who sees them as involving too much time and too many uncertainties, as well as possible alteration of the Unitas program in unacceptable ways.

After receiving funds for 1979, Unitas resumed a full operating schedule and new personnel were brought it. In February, a second full-time B.A.-level social worker, Rosalie, was hired mainly to do outreach family therapy. However, like Garcia, her male counterpart, she also participated in many other aspects of the program.

At the same time, Lynn Stekas, an MSW social worker, was hired as full-time administrator of the program. Her six years of social work experience prior to joining Unitas involved casework, group and community outreach counseling, coordinating and supervising group work programs, and supervising social-work students for Catholic Charities. After completing an MSW at Hunter College (CUNY) in 1977 she worked in administrative positions. As coordinator of a youth program for Catholic Charities, she developed and managed a sports league for 2,000 children and 200 adult volunteers in Queens. She was also responsible for writing, administering and evaluating a Youth Board contract for a Catholic parish. Her experience also includes years of work as a teenager in charge of all the bookkeeping for her father's small business. Stekas also points to her marriage to a former accountant (turned social worker) as helpful in administering Unitas.

Stekas' Unitas responsibilities have primarily entailed overseeing all administrative functions of the agency but, as a trained therapist, she has also become involved in other aspects of the program. She supervises several social-work students training at Unitas, runs a weekly young women's group and a weekly group of young men, all of whom are now or are about to be in college. The newly created position which Stekas holds brings with it opportunities for her to expand Unitas programming in significant ways, such as developing the institutional ties and the therapy groups just described. But Stekas' energies have perforce been focused on the management of Unitas and on trying to raise funds to keep the agency running.

The above historical sketch of Unitas makes clear how Eismann and Unitas are bound together as concept, program, and organization. Edward P. Eismann was born in New York City in 1932 to German-Irish parents. He was educated in the local public schools in New York City. Although his family, which included his parents and sister, did retain some aspects of German culture, Eismann describes his background as being "simply American." Perhaps this explains Eismann's implicit encouragement of cultural assimilation by requiring English to be spoken, by deemphasizing cultural ties, and by preparing Unitas members to enter the mainstream of middle-class American structure.

Since both his parents worked, Eismann became independent at an early age, developing his imagination and creativity. He recalls forming a restaurant in his cellar, where he would serve his father, and opening an animal hospital in his home where he cared for stray cats and dogs. This quality of providing service is continually reflected in his life.

Eismann points to his adolescent years in Brooklyn as especially significant in forming his present philosophy. He describes those years as very lonely, since he never had a sense of belonging to any group outside the family.

> One of the things I prayed so much for were friendships with other kids, but somehow I did not have the confidence in myself that other kids would like me.

He could not assert himself with others, was shy with girls, and wary of the gangs in his neighborhood. One of the reasons that Eismann formed Unitas may have been to enable other children to avoid the same sense of loneliness that he experienced.

> I think, "What have I done?" I have created a lot of friends of kids. I have created a group.

Eismann feels that as a child he was lacking an adult outside the family upon whom he could rely and with whom he could feel comfortable. He was still very young when he decided that he wanted to become that adult for other children. For this reason, he decided to become a priest -- priests were, to his knowledge, the only people offering direct helping service to children and the neighborhood. He viewed teachers, who were in fact important in forming his self-image, merely as people who imparted information. Through the sacrament of Penance, Eismann could go to a priest and have an intimate dialogue; however, in the confessional booth he was assumed guilty, evaluated, judged, and scolded. "That is all

I needed when I was a guilt-ridden kid," he reflects.

Eismann was actively involved in church functions. During his teen years, he taught Sunday School and Wednesday-afternoon released-time religion classes at the local church. He also played organ at masses and headed a children's choir. Eismann did two years of undergraduate study at St. John's University in Brooklyn where his long-time love of music flourished. In high school, he played the piano in the Glee Club and helped create music groups for youngsters. He played the piccolo and the flute in the school band and as a member of a swing band performed at weddings and receptions. Today, Eismann is a classical organist and pianist, although he has not applied these talents within Unitas.

At St. John's University he became more philosophical and experienced a growing sense of dissatisfaction with music alone.

> I wanted whatever I did to be worth something eternal and infinite. I did not want my life to be meaningless. I wanted to be a person who dealt with others in a way that was different from what I had experienced.

With this in mind, Eismann transferred to a seminary college in Massachusetts operated by the Congregation of Holy Cross. As a religious order the congregation emphasized the values of silence, prayer, and a varied, active ministry. He graduated and was admitted to the order's novitiate. Ordination consisted of a four-year graduate program. Eismann spent his novitiate year in Bennington, Vermont, and for the next four years, 1954-1958, he attended Holy Cross Theological College at the Catholic University of America in Washington, D.C. During this time, Eismann worked part-time with a group of black children from the Washington slums, incarcerated youth in a detention center, the mentally ill in a federal hospital, and neglected children in a group home.

At the end of his third year, Eismann began to have doubts about being ordained. He realized that he did not want a formation exclusively founded on theology, but one that integrated an understanding of human relations as well, which was the aspect of the priesthood that had initially attracted him. Eismann wanted to learn more about people and understand them better, to give them "helpful service built on knowledge, not just impulse." He left Theological College five months before ordination, receiving a one year's indult of exclaustration from Rome. During this year, 1957, he worked in a Boy's Home, where he received room and board, and attended the School of Social Work of Catholic Univeristy of America, paid for by the Congregation. For a time he entered Freudian analysis but, in keeping with his desire to move away from introspection toward interaction, he found the experience dissatisfying. In 1959 Eismann received an MSW degree from Catholic University.

Eismann never returned for ordination, but has remained faithful to the Catholic Church. He stresses the importance of Judeo-Christian underpinnings in his development and present sense of self. However, he feels that there are many ways to worship in addition to the ways of a traditional church, such as by simply gathering together people and letting leaders naturally emerge who can assist people to express and share their religious sentiment among themselves in a natural community. This is, in his words, "everything Unitas is."

After graduation from the School of Social Work, Eismann returned to New York to work for Catholic Charities in a child guidance clinic from 1961 to 1965. For six months during this period Eismann was in Sullivanian analysis, after which he turned to Adlerian analysis, the latter having a profound effect on his views of therapy and mental health. He became increasingly dissatisfied with an analytic approach to therapy, although he acknowledges its contribution to his personal growth. One feature which impressed him was that his Adlerian analyst was a good listener and was not opinionated. This attracted him since the major help figures in his past, priests and teachers, seemed to pass judgment freely. Eventually Eismann entered group therapy, an experience which exerted an influence on the creation of Unitas in that "what people could give to each other was reinforced in my own group experience."

In the summer of 1963 Eismann traveled to Mexico City where he cared for a young boy and attended the Instituto Norteamericano to learn Spanish. The following summer he worked in Argentina and Chile in a self-help village project. Eismann then returned to school to obtain a doctorate in clinical social work from Smith College, in a conjoint plan with Harvard University. After receiving a Ph.D. in 1967, he traveled around the United States for two months and decided that he wanted to settle down in a lifetime career. He was torn between his family in New York and his desire to work in Hull House in Chicago. After hearing about the Bronx community mental health center and its new thrust in helping people, Eismann returned to New York and began working there. He pursued post-doctoral training at the Alfred Adler Psychoanalytic Institute in New York, which stressed interpersonal relations and he received that Institute's diploma in 1972.

In the early 1970's, Eismann felt that he would like to have a more permanent relation with a child, instead of dealing with children throughout the day and then having them return to their real mothers and fathers at day's end. Eismann approached Catholic Charities about adopting a child, and within six months

Eismann was given Tom, a nine-year-old boy. Tom was born in the Bronx, was abandoned by his mother, and brought to Catholic Charities by his father. After that, the child had been in and out of foster homes. In 1974, within a year after receiving him, Eismann legally adopted Tom. Eismann and his son now share an apartment in the Parkchester section of the Bronx. Tom is a high school student and an active symbolic parent in Unitas.

In terms of family life for himself, Eismann says that his lifestyle does not necessarily exclude marriage. Unitas is his entire life, but Eismann does not feel than an emotional involvement would diminish his commitment to the program. It is difficult, though not impossible, to imagine Ed Eismann involved in other activities with the intense devotion that characterizes his concern for Unitas. However, in tracing his personal development, we find that such seriousness of purpose and zeal have been hallmarks of Eismann's work. His clarity of vision coupled with dogged hard work have enabled Unitas to develop as carefully as it has. Unitas has survived and flourished through a period of community deterioration, cutbacks in funding, staff shortages and turnovers, and upheavals in the community mental health field. In large part we must attribute its growth to the dedication and abilities of its founder, Edward P. Eismann.

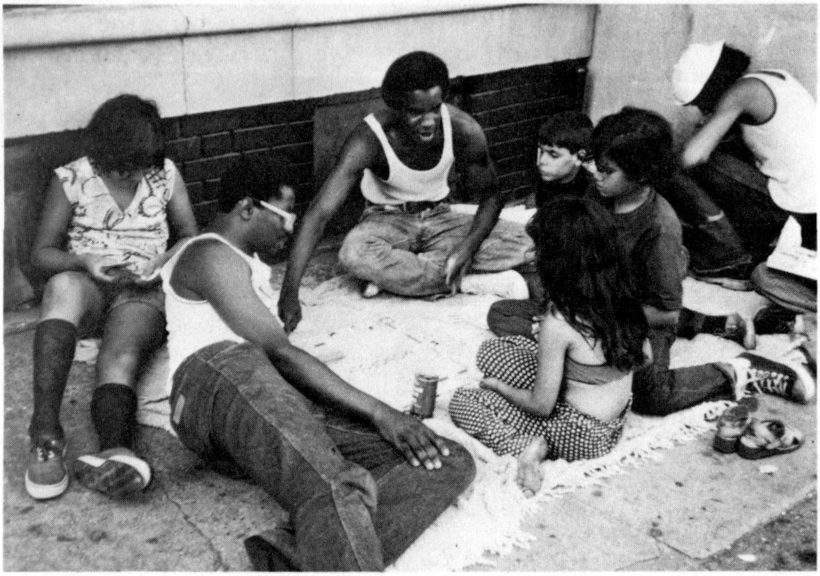

PLATE 6. "In Unitas children learn to absorb losing as well as enjoy winning; develop ever increasing levels of socialization; develop cooperation as well as autonomy."

V

SOCIAL ORGANIZATION

As in a family, so in Unitas individuals receive encouragement and support for their dependency. In the context of kinship, dependency generally implies inequality, the dependent one subordinate to a superior, powerful relative. In the natural family, the parents have power over the children, and the older children often hold sway over their younger siblings. Aunts and uncles, though clearly not the mothers and fathers of the nuclear unit, are recognized as parental or potential equivalents. Power, then, within the family unit, reflects age and kinship role, which often correspond. The structure of Unitas encourages this kind of dependency and hierarchy, with power assigned according to age and family connection, albeit a created, symbolic one.

Since children are usually cared for and socialized by their biological families, the justification for the creation of an elaborate symbolic family structure needs to be discussed further. Eismann's view is that a great number of actual families in poverty stricken, ghetto areas "are so disrupted and disorganized that they are virtually inaccessible to change through family treatment." Whether this is indeed true is not the issue here, although the problem is certainly an important one. Unitas begins with the premise that traditional family therapy intervention in disrupted families is, at best, minimally effective. According to Eismann, the climate of actual family life for many families in ghetto circumstances may be psychologically damaging for all involved.

Without addressing himself to the specific social and economic causes of this unhealthy situation, Eismann charges Unitas with the awesome task of resocializing in healthy ways youth who have been psychologically hurt by their families. He states that

> ...the troubled kids need mothers and fathers. This means that they didn't get enough of their parents.

> If a mother is raising ten kids, maybe alone, then she has a lot to do and perhaps can't give enough to each of her children. When a kid comes to us angry, we don't smack the kid in the head. He probably gets enough of that. There are other ways.

Eismann portrays an angry, overburdened single mother without healthy options in her life. It is the family system which is unhealthy and in need of fundamental change, not simply the child-rearing behavior of the mother. The social system in which she operates, however, is not readily amenable to improvement.

Psychological health involves people helping, caring for, and controlling each other, as well as sharing their thoughts and feelings. When people are able to nourish one another, then they are like the members of one family, a healthy family. Ironically, this kind of nourishing or healing does not often take place in real families in which the parents are emotionally unavailable to help their children. Such is the situation which prevails to a large extent in the South Bronx. The justification, then, for working with symbolic families lies in the need of children who are in an unhealthy, dysfunctional real family structure to receive adequate parenting elsewhere. Unitas claims to provide such a healthy surrogate structure.

Unitas is conceived as "one big family made up of little families." All participants in Unitas become members of a small symbolic family. Together, these symbolic families form an extended family. Authority resides with the grandfather, the oldest and most powerful family member. There is only one grandfather; there is no grandmother in the Unitas family model. Moving downward through the generations, there are mothers and fathers, structurally equal to one another who are the heads of the small Unitas family units. Their responsibility is to care for their Unitas children, who are divided into older children and less responsible younger children. Each family may have one or more aunts and uncles. Older than children, but not ready to be parents, aunts and uncles are regarded as parents-in-training; it is expected that they will move into symbolic parent positions quickly.

Unlike biological families, Unitas families rarely extend formal kinship terminology beyond the immediate members. Even within the small family unit, not all kinship ties are recognized. When either addressing or referring to a Unitas mother or father of another family, a parent does not use a sister, brother, or in-law term. Sibling relationships exist only in the child generation. Only children have brothers and sisters; their "parents" do not. Similarly, while there are Unitas parents, there are no Unitas spouses. Unitas does not recognize symbolic marital ties, and there are no symbolic husbands and wives. The Unitas family members use only first names in speaking to or about the others.

An exception to this is the use of the terms cousin, sister, and brother in the child generation. Cousin and sibling terms are used by Eismann when he asks a child from one family to interact with another child in the same family or in a different Unitas family. This serves two functions. First, it relieves Eismann of the burden of having to remember the hundreds of names of Unitas children. Second and more importantly, it reinforces the ties that Unitas children have as symbolic family members to one another. The focus here, as it is in much of the Unitas structure, is on the bonding between children and their peers, facilitated by the symbolic parents.

At the center of Unitas are the teenagers acting in the roles of mothers and fathers. Unitas mothers and fathers fall into two main groups: those who have been in Unitas for several years and have proven their abilities and commitment, and those who are relatively new to Unitas and are still being tested and trained. As a group, the Unitas parents form the backbone of the program; without them, there would be no program as it now exists.

In 1979 five teenagers could be singled out as wielding greater power in Unitas than their contemporaries. These five had more contact with the children, with Eismann, and with other Unitas administrators than other teens. They acted as mediators between other teenagers in the program and the administration, and as the interpreters and translators of Unitas policy to the children. Through the years this number has shifted, but since its beginnings Unitas has always had a group of dedicated, influential teenagers. In this year, we meet Juan, George, Richard, Carlos, and Terry. There are a number of features which these teens share, not the least of which is their true-believer dedication to Unitas, as both an organization and a way of life.

As a group, these five tend to be closer to Unitas children and their families than other teenagers. This closeness, observable in the ways they talk to and touch the children, and the frequency of their contacts with children and their real families, as well as the concern they show for their well-being, comes from the years of Unitas training in child development and behavior. We can easily trace the values underlying the behaviors of these symbolic parents toward their children and each other to Unitas' teachings. Examples will serve to illustrate the differences in behaviors between the experienced teens and the novices.

It is a Thursday afternoon in April 1979. At 3:15 small children begin to enter the St. Athanasius gym to participate in the Unitas circle. Eismann greets each child at the door, asking which family he or she is in. Eismann explains that this practice maintains order, sets the mood of the gathering, and reinforces the children's commitment to the symbolic family.

A smile, a gentle greeting, and often a warm touch welcomes each child as he or she arrives at George's family. George is 21 years old, black, lives at home with his parents, and is about to graduate from high school and begin college. "Hello Darlene, how was your day? Nice to see you." "Hey, Leo, hello. Come sit down." George draws the children one by one into his caring nest. Within ten minutes, there are perhaps fifteen black and Hispanic girls and boys assembled around George, who now has Sara on his lap and an arm around Greg, a sad looking boy of nine. George never ceases to interact with the children, intently watching and responding to their activities. When they are gathered he asks them to arrange themselves, seated, in a circle, so that they can play a game. It takes a couple of minutes, a bit of verbal and physical nudging, and the enlistment of the older children's assistance but the circle gets formed without George ever raising his voice. The game involves one person in the family trying to name the other members of the family. Several of the children are anxious to show their skill. Henry, a boy of 10, names perhaps half the children. When he cannot remember a name, George urges him to ask the person directly what his name is. Other children are encouraged to help Henry in this task but not to tell him the name. Most of the children comply; a few cannot resist whispering the name, but this is mostly ignored by George and, following his lead, by the other family members.

Now it's José's turn. When he gets to Leo, the only excessively overweight boy in the family, José calls out "Fatso." The children laugh, as José apparently intended. Without hesitation, George mildly but clearly and publicly reprimands José and tells him the correct name to use. As soon as George speaks, the snickering stops.

This contrasts with the conduct of Jesus, a Unitas parent like George, but without George's degree of commitment or incorporation of Unitas philosophy, and without George's gentle control over himself and the children. Jesus arrives a few minutes late at his family's usual location in the Unitas circle on this Thursday. He hurries in and heads immediately to Howard, his friend from the streets, also a father in another family, to say hello. Juan, the more experienced and responsible father in this family, frowns, showing his displeasure at his co-parent's actions. He briefly mentions Jesus' lateness and stopover at Howard's family. Jesus, however, directs his attention toward a couple of the boys in his family who are nearby, anxious to be with him. He cannot resist this opportunity to avoid Juan's criticism. He tousles the back of one boy's hair, pushing his head forward as he does it. As the boy stumbles forward, laughing and clearly enjoying the attention, Jesus turns toward his friend, Johnny, and lunges for his legs, startling the boy but nothing more. They are all laughing now, and although there has clearly been positive interaction between these boys and their surrogate father, one wonders inevitably about the therapeutic value of these actions. Therapy does not seem to be foremost on Jesus' mind at the moment. Soon, however, Jesus is seated with his family as they prepare for the weekly Unitas circle. The children, Robbie and Johnny, are by his side, now joined by Frank, who is busily chatting about a television program he had seen the night before. Two girls standing nearby greet Jesus shyly and Jesus says hello to them but makes no effort to bring them into the circle. The girls drift to a spot near Juan and sit down.

George has been coming to Unitas for nearly six years, since he was fifteen years old. In addition to being a symbolic father in the Unitas family, George tutors children in reading, does therapeutic work with local families, meets individually with troubled children, works in art therapy, does group counselling, plans group outings, and supervises youth workers. He is proud of the work he does in Unitas, of his commitment to the program and of the changes he has experienced personally. "In 1974, I was making the transition from child to worker," he explains. "I grew up in the program. In high school I was quiet and never spoke to anyone. Then, Carlos and I started talking to each other. That's how I got here."

The talking that George refers to is not the kind of verbal badinage that we routinely hear from, say, Jesus. Rather, the speech is highly explicit in form and intention; its stated and understood purpose being to facilitate communication between the speakers. In training sessions, the teenagers, motivated in varying degrees by their desires to harmonize with other teens and workers and to handle the difficult children more effectively, learn communication skills along with therapeutic techniques. The two cannot easily be separated, however, since effective communication -- verbal and non-verbal -- is crucial to effective healing. The problem, as George explains it, is to "get the kids to interact with each other," and this cannot be done by explaining it to them. "They cannot grasp it, they have to experience it." George no longer feels that there is a fundamental distinction between his behavior outside and his behavior within the Unitas context.

Jesus, when asked about these issues, hesitates and falters, not knowing how to respond. He agrees that communication is superior to hitting as a way of handling a difficult situation. But Jesus does not speak with the same commitment and understanding that one hears from George. Observing Jesus playing during the recreation hour of the family circle meeting on this Thursday, we see him involved in a basketball game with five other boys, all but one of whom are in their teens. On the sidelines stand two boys, perhaps nine years old, watching the game. It is a Unitas uncle, not Jesus, a Unitas father, who invited them to join the game. As part of their training, Eismann insists that the teenagers not confuse their recreational work with the children with their own amusement. The teens are not, he stresses, there to play their own games; they are at Unitas to work. Evidently, Jesus has not learned this lesson well.

Jesus has no regular responsibilities in Unitas the way that George does, but then he has only been in the program for eight months. During the last summer, he moved to Fox Street from a different section of the South Bronx. During that summer Jesus saw people playing on the street during the afternoons. Not working, with no money and only a few friends, Jesus found himself lured by the activity he watched. One day in August, he left his house determined to find out how to participate. The first person he met was Juan who took Jesus under his wing, introduced him to others, and helped him feel comfortable.

Jesus can be understood perhaps as a young George in the sense that he is the age George was when he first came to Unitas, and, at least by his interest and attendance, he is as dedicated to the program. Also, both George and Jesus were motivated at first by their loneliness and the need to participate in a group. Perhaps time and training -- and with these, maturity -- will overcome Jesus' lack of skills and sensitivity, and develop in him a genuine commitment to Unitas goals.

Incorporation into the Unitas hierarchy is slow, often requiring years for a teenager to be given or to take a place of authority in the structure. We have identified two routes toward incorporation. One can start out as a child in Unitas and eventually take on greater responsibilities within the family and the organization. This was how Richard and Carlos, for example, joined Unitas. A second route is to join Unitas as a teenager and, through commitment, work, and the desire and ability to fit in, be accepted. Juan, Terry, and Neil followed this approach. This is the faster but perhaps more difficult of the two avenues into the inner circle because it requires that an already formed teenager, new to the organization, prove his or her ability to do the work well and to fit into the value system and with the other workers of the organization.

Until the summer of 1977, there was what the teens called a "hot seat." Eismann would first interview the new teenager in front of the group and then the group would interview him with Eismann present. The person would be asked about his or her interests, experiences with children, and ability to speak in a large group. This procedure is no longer followed in large part because of the internal restructuring of Unitas. In the past there was no separate core of teenagers hired as summer workers as there are now. Teenagers had to serve in Unitas during the winter to prove themselves and to make friendships with other teens. The "hot seat" served as a test administered by the Unitas upper echelon to worthy novices. Now, summer workers are provided with the same work experience as the teens in the past but without the burden of going on "trial." Most temporary summer teens view Unitas as an agency in which they are placed to work for an hourly wage. For those teens dedicated to the program, there is still the element of testing but it is now diluted by the presence of many uncommitted youth, a fact which disturbs many of the more devoted Unitas workers.

Not all teenagers who are assigned to Unitas, however, are allowed to remain in the program. In 1979, six summer workers were asked to leave and their transfers to other work sites arranged. The main reason given for the transfer was the inability of these teenagers to interact with others. They were either too shy or too marginal, because of their own anger or lack of interest. Of note is that five of the six dismissed teenagers were girls; the sixth, a male, was transferred out of Unitas on the first day because he was too young, not because of personal difficulties. Perhaps it was chance that only females were asked to leave Unitas during that summer, but most likely it was not. The shyness that was cited as the reason for the transfer of two Puerto Rican girls is a characteristic personality trait of many Hispanic females. Two black girls, friends who tended to stay by themselves on the street, were asked to leave in part because of complaints from other teenagers who observed that these girls had "an attitude." Other teenagers, males, were also mentioned as being only marginally acceptable, but none were asked to leave. They remain, according to Eismann, because, although they may be too young and "dull," they are known in Unitas, and are neighborhood kids. "If they came to me now," claims Eismann, "I'd probably have them reassigned." Unitas will not go out of its way to accept children or teenagers from outside of the community. They are striving to build on local turf, to incorporate this into Unitas' daily functioning. In 1980, to avoid earlier problems, teenagers deemed unacceptable were weeded out in interviews before they began to work in the program.

The Unitas circle illustrates another feature which can be used to measure differences between one symbolic parent and another: attractiveness of the parent to the children. Through their actions, the teens communicate to the children different degrees of interest in them and their activities. It is this natural attractiveness which Unitas uses to establish symbolic families. Children are not assigned to a family when they enter Unitas. They spend time in a family that appeals to them and into which they are welcome. If they choose, they may switch families. It is not uncommon, also, to find a child who has one parent in one family and a second parent in a different family.

The use of natural attraction sometimes leads to situations which may be embarrassing to teenagers. During the summer of 1979, when time to organize and implement the program was severely limited, Eismann decided to let the established families select new teenagers, who had been assigned to Unitas, to serve as aunts and uncles in their symbolic families. The means to do this -- lining up teenagers outside, at the end of a circle meeting, and having family groups choose their favorites -- emphasized individual differences and public display. As noted earlier, Unitas does not extend the same kind of unconditional welcome to its new teenage workers as it does to its children. They must work hard and make themselves attractive to other teenagers and to children in order to succeed.

One way to quantify this attractiveness is to look at the number of children who are in the families of the teenagers. We would expect that the more children in a teenager's family, the greater that teenager's appeal. Further refining measures of a teenager's appeal are, at best, a difficult task. We might hypothesize that a teenager's attractiveness to children would consist of a combination of his or her personal characteristics, including physical attributes, commitment to the children's needs, and skills in fulfilling these needs. Also, bound to influence at least some children is their sense of which teenagers have been informally designated as leaders by Eismann. As an initial measure, we are considering the number of children in a teen parent's family as a broad measure of attractiveness, encompassing the finer indicators mentioned above.

In this study, two methods -- Unitas parent information, from roll books and from questioning of parents, and information from questioning of children -- were used to learn the structure of family units. Once we learned the structure, we added up the numbers of children per family and per "parent." What about families in which there are more than one Unitas parent? We handled this by asking children for the names of all their Unitas parents, and by asking each Unitas parent to name all the members of his or her families. Not all "parents" named all the children in their family; they generally provided the names of only those children for whom they are responsible. Family structures could then be combined to learn the total number of children per family. This would not, however, offer adequate information concerning the appeal of one particular teen "parent" versus another. Thus, the only method that proved useful in this pursuit was the second, the questioning of each child about his or her Unitas parent(s).

The size of the teenagers' Unitas families as reflected in the children's naming of their symbolic parents indicates, though imperfectly, their relative positions in the Unitas hierarchy. For this analysis, we designated three groups of Unitas workers: (1) Administrative workers and professional trainees. Administrative workers include paid full-time staff whether they are working primarily as therapists or administrators. It does not include experienced workers who, though they may work at Unitas full-time, were not specifically brought into the agency to fill a particular employment slot. (2) Inner-circle workers. These are the workers who make up the core group of Unitas. In 1979, each of the five in this group had been involved in the program since 1976, and tended to be older than the other teens, ranging in age from 17 to 21. (3) Teen workers. This category includes both "up-and-coming inner-circle" workers and marginal teen workers -- the least experienced and least committed workers at Unitas. The latter category includes teenagers who were assigned to Unitas by the Youth Employment Program for summer jobs and who never returned after August, as well as teenagers who continue to participate in Unitas but tend to remain peripheral to it.

We find that the five core workers had larger Unitas family groups than other workers. They averaged ten children each. Two of the workers in this group, Juan and Terry, had surprisingly low numbers, with only four and six children each, respectively. Closer examination of the data reveals, however, that there are sound reasons in each case for this finding. During the summer, Juan worked more as a supervisor and coordinator than as a counselor to the children. He had the responsibility of managing the lunch crew to assure that the children received lunches every day and that these lunches were cleaned up. Thus, he rarely ate with the children or stayed with them before or after their lunch. Also, Juan generally took more of an interest in the other teens, making sure that they were doing their jobs well, than in working directly with the children. Had he not incorporated the Unitas values and policies so well, he would not have been allowed such managerial license to translate and interpret Unitas philosophy to his contemporaries. It is not unusual to hear Eismann talk of Juan's special sensitivity and expression. Juan's position is more one of middle-management than of worker.

Terry, Juan's girlfriend since before coming to Unitas, also occupies a special position in Unitas. Unlike other Puerto Rican girls who participate in the program, Terry is not nor was she ever shy. Eismann describes her as "the brain and she can sound cold." He suggests that "she could learn to be more mellow and affectionate." But like Juan, Terry articulates Unitas philosophy well and adamantly, never hesitating to interpret Eismann's teachings to other teens. It is perhaps because of this ability that Terry has become one of Eismann's favorites. Terry's outspokenness and coldness, coupled with her considerable time commitment to her college work -- she is preparing to attend law school -- account for her lack of a strong following among the children.

Compared to the average family size of 10 for the inner-circle teens, the "up-and-coming" teenagers averaged 6.3 children in their symbolic families during the summer, and the "marginal teen workers" averaged only 2.2 children each. To the extent that the numbers accurately reflect the commitment to and involvement in Unitas, this appeal quotient works well, with the inner-circle workers averaging more children than either of the teen worker categories. In short, with few exceptions, the more involved the teenager, the greater will be his or her popularity among the children, that is, the more attractive he or she will be.

We should note that the involvement of the workers goes beyond economic concerns. During the 1979 summer program, all the teen workers were paid the same hourly wage. In 1980, college students were paid $150 per week through the Summer Work Training Program, considerably more than the $110 per week paid to high school students. As in any group, some workers fit well into the Unitas structure and others did not, regardless of their salaries. We cannot, therefore, attribute differences in participation to differences in subsequent rewards for labor. The zealousness with which many of the teens and other workers devote themselves to Unitas helps explain Unitas' ability to run year after year on a shoestring budget.

Three related questions might well be asked here. First, why do some teenagers succeed in Unitas while others do not? What qualities characterize inner-circle workers and up-and-coming teen workers, distinguishing them from marginal teen workers and teens who have been asked to leave the program? Second, what is it about Unitas, the teens, or both, which fosters the hard work and devotion which we observe, and without which the program could not continue? And third, what is the process of moving from up-and-coming teen status to inner-circle status? Each of these questions concerns the maintenance of the hierarchy of workers in Unitas and it is this to which we now turn our attention.

Unitas offers teenagers friendships and the skills necessary to develop and keep them. When we asked teenage workers to tell the story of how they first came to Unitas, several themes emerged. Some marginal youth workers, those assigned to Unitas by the Youth Employment Program to work for the summer, were not personally motivated to join Unitas. They came to Unitas as a job, only in a few instances reporting that they found the work satisfying. None of the teenagers in this category stayed in Unitas beyond the summer. Other marginal teenagers, those with longer histories in Unitas and greater commitment to the program, were often attracted for reasons having little to do with the primary substance of the program. Peter, for example, entered Unitas four years ago, when he was twelve years old. He has been coming regularly ever since, participating in both the winter and summer programs. He is now an uncle in Richard's family. This is significant because first, Peter is old enough to be a Unitas father (the minimum age for symbolic parenthood is fifteen; Peter is now sixteen) and second, he entered Unitas at the same time as or even earlier than other teenagers who have since moved into symbolic parent roles. Peter responds to the questions, "What was your first experience with Unitas? What attracted you to Unitas?" as follows:

> George and Richard told me about it. They told me that there would be a lot of sports and other stuff, that I would have to go through routines, like meetings, that there would be a lot of girls. So I said, "All right! Let me go!" That was enough.

When asked why he stuck with it, Peter responds,

> "Because of the girls and the sports."

Peter, however, does feel connected to other teenagers in Unitas, especially to Jimmy, a boy from the block where he lives whom he knew before he came into the program. Unlike inner-circle workers, who talk of how they slowly developed friendships with other teenagers whom they met in Unitas, Peter has a hard time distinguishing one friendship within Unitas from another, claiming that the teenagers are "all the same, all my friends," with the exception of Jimmy, whom he names as a closer friend.

Unitas has been influential in Peter's life, however, apart from providing him with sports and girls. In talking of a problem that he and Jimmy were having he says that:

> We talked about it. I wouldn't have done it if it weren't for Unitas. Usually if a friend does something against you, you strike him out and put him down as an enemy, but here we learn to give a second chance, to see his point of view.

Peter did not like Unitas at all when he first came. He didn't like sitting on the floor or on the street, the meetings were boring and seemed interminable, the children were very hard to handle and, finally, he couldn't accept the Unitas style of problem-solving which relied on talking rather than directly acting, usually in physical ways. Struggle is the term Peter chooses to describe the time he has spent in Unitas, especially to solve problems.

In spite of his seniority in Unitas -- both in terms of age and the length of time involved -- Peter must be classified as a marginal teen worker. He cares for only one child in his symbolic family, has created no strong bonds in Unitas with other teens, and has taken on no responsibilities which might serve to create such connections. Perhaps at the base of this is his lack of commitment to Unitas. It is not simply that Peter does not understand the Unitas teachings. His description of the change he has experienced in his methods of resolving conflict with his close friend Jimmy illustrates that he has incorporated some of the program's philosophy. It is, rather, that he has not accepted Unitas as a crucial part of his life, the *nexus* of his social activities and friendships, the place where he feels most connected and the most growth.

Contrast Peter with Neil, a black teenager two years older, now eighteen, who has been in Unitas for a little over one year. Neil heard about Unitas from Juan whom he knew from the high school where they were both students. Neil does not, nor has he ever, lived in the South Bronx. He lives with his mother in the north central area of the Bronx, a residential section that has, until recently, been predominantly Jewish and Irish. After being told about Unitas, and especially about Doc, numerous times, Neil decided to see what the experience would be like. What attracted him was not the recreational aspects of the program or the girls he would meet but the relationships that Juan had described. Neil describes his first experiences with Unitas:

> I was in awe. I had been thinking about working in a center or something to occupy my free time, but I wanted it to be meaningful, something where I could teach a kid or help the kid instead of just being an instructor and give out equipment to a kid and say, "Sign your name and bring it back when you're finished" or something like that. I saw that there were a lot of things happening here...by some of the ways things were set up with kids being in families -- some of the people being considered mothers and fathers and uncles and aunts. It shows a lot of responsibility because of the way things were taken care of, with a child considering you as a father or a mother. There would be a lot of responsibilities to that child and other children in the family. You would have to be there with them. It was more of a personal relationship to the kids instead of being just a figure of authority.

Besides being attracted by the relationship that he believes he could establish with the children, Neil describes ways in which he thought his friendships with other teenagers could be deepened. He also looked forward to sharing the other teenagers' dedication:

> I guess I had only seen the other teenagers playing basketball, just seeing them in school or at a friend's house, talking about sports or something. There was more to them than just that. Not the fact that there was just more to them but for them to have the dedication to being in Unitas! That's what I saw. That, most of all, it would take a lot of self-dedication.

Having established that inner-circle workers are not distinguishable from other teen workers on the basis of age or length of time involved in the program, we turn to other factors in determining who will be successful in the program and who will not. There are three related features which characterize the most successful teenagers: First, their perceptions of Unitas and their dedication to the program and its philosophy; second, the route by which they entered the program; and third, their friendship network in Unitas. Earlier in this chapter we mentioned various appeals that Unitas has held for teenagers and the differing degrees of commitment that followed. We intimated that those who were initially attracted to Unitas by its philosophy were more likely to rise in the hierarchy. This, of course, comes as no surprise. It stands to reason that accurate perceptions both of the program and their potential roles and growth within it would lead teenagers to successful participation. In this respect, the Unitas hierarchical structure is based more on the identification of appropriate teenage participants than on the creation of them.

This leads us to the second feature characterizing successful teenagers related to the question: Do successful teenage workers come into Unitas in a way different from more marginal workers? There are various routes or social networks into Unitas: personal contact, therapeutic contact, and institutional contact. Personal contact refers to those associations with Unitas that originated in personal ties with Eismann. These ties are often institutionally based, such as when a school principal who knows of Eismann's work refers a teacher to Unitas. Institutional contact refers to communications based primarily on institutional rather than personal relations. Included in this category are Eismann's contacts with government agencies which assign otherwise unknown teenagers to work. Although some teenagers were paid through institutions such as the Youth Employment Program, only those teenagers whose first contact with Unitas was established via this route are included here. None of the teenagers assigned in this way participate regularly in Unitas, although two in this category, now both in college, have expressed interest in returning to work on a salaried basis during the summer. Therapeutic contact refers to relationships established by Eismann, usually directly, but sometimes through a mental health worker, with a child or teenager. Only two inner-circle workers, Richard and Carlos, entered Unitas in this manner. The other inner-circle workers were brought into Unitas initially by one of these workers. The point, however, is that workers in the inner-circle, and those in the process of being accepted into that group, entered and are entering Unitas only through one route, through therapeutic contact.

Richard has been in Unitas since 1967, when he was eight years old. He was a shy child, by his own description, and did not readily join in the street games on Fox Street. He did, however, hang around the outskirts of the group. He talks with some pleasure of the attention he received now and then from Eismann and the art therapist. The turning point came when Richard was thirteen. He had just been fired from a job at a hardware store and so had time to spare. Eismann invited him to the local community mental health center, where he met Mr. Paul, a teacher in a local school, who had been working with Eismann for several years. Richard began to come regularly, to help Mr. Paul with a group of children. At the same time, in Richard's words,

> "I also went over to the settlement house. Also Doc and I would sit in his car and talk for hours, and became friends...The process took about four years. Doc had to convince me."

Although Richard often talks as if he has spent most of his life in Unitas, his real involvement in the program only truly begins, according to his description, when he reaches his early teens. Richard speaks of the importance of not only "Doc" in his life at that time, but of Henry and Jose, then the best known, most powerful teenagers in Unitas. And, from his earliest association with Unitas, Richard identifies only with those doing the therapy or the helping -- Mr. Paul, Doc, and later the older teenagers -- than with those being helped.

Carlos' involvement in Unitas begins somewhat differently, but is also characterized by initial reluctance. Unlike Richard, Carlos was specifically referred to Unitas first by a teacher and later by a guidance counselor. Carlos is now 22 years old, working full-time as a superintendent of a building, but still finds time to come to Unitas with regularity. He tells the story of how he first became involved in Unitas:

> I used to not talk in school. I used to be a quiet boy. The teacher told Doc about me. We three sat down to meet. Doc invited me to Unitas but I didn't go because, first, I didn't know what it was all about and, second, I didn't go places. So he found me in the park, in school. He took me to the mental health center and I said, "This is a place for nutty people." I saw kids and I said, "Now I'm a nut, in a weird place!" We sat in Doc's office and talked. He told me to come back but I didn't show up again. A couple of weeks later Doc came to my house and invited me again and I never showed up. This went on for about a year.
>
> Then, in junior high school, I was a terrible boy in school, attendance-wise. I was still quiet. I didn't

> stay in school. I'd go home. The guidance counselor told Doc about me. Doc came to my house to make a home visit, like he does now. But I still wouldn't go to the mental health center. They were going to send me to a children's home. Doc gave me a choice, to go to school or be sent away.

Eismann talks of sometimes anticipating what would probably happen to a child. He would present the child with the choices, as though they were not in the future but in the present, thus giving the child a clear sense of his options while he was still in a position to make decisions. In Carlos' case, the threat of being sent away to a children's home was not imminent, but Eismann used this to get him "on the right track" before the threat became real. Carlos, responding to the clear message delivered by Eismann, decided to return to school. He continues:

> I would spend the morning in school and the afternoon in the mental health center. Mr. Paul, a teacher, was tutoring me. My sister was in his class so I knew about him. I was in eighth grade at the time...Difference now was that now it was my school. I thought I'd get marked absent if I didn't go. I graduated by some miracle! Doc arranged it.

Indeed, Eismann had arranged with the guidance counselor and a health teacher for Carlos to follow the unorthodox route of attending school in the morning only and to be marked present for the day. Each afternoon Carlos would be tutored individually by Mr. Paul at the community mental health center. Once Carlos graduated, he continued to go to Unitas, but he was no longer being tutored. He was in high school and, by his own account, had good grades. In 1974, when he was in tenth grade, Carlos' father died, throwing him into confusion. He decided to turn to Eismann for help.

> I went to Doc and asked for a job. Doc said, "Sure but you've got to be tested. You have to come to the center to be interviewed by all the teenagers and if they like you, you can stay, and if they don't...Oh well." I had to go through an initiation, that's what we call it now. I said, "This program is not all that bad," so I decided to try it. I went to the initiation at the center. They asked me all sorts of questions. I talked about school, where I'm from. Doc said I'd have to work for a month first as a volunteer before I could get paid. I came on Thursday afternoon to St. Athanasius.

Carlos volunteered for a time, attending the Thursday circles regularly as well as spending time at the community mental health center, talking with other teens, working in the wood workshop that Eismann had established in an empty basement office.

Both Carlos and Richard speak of their early resistance to Unitas and their gradual seduction into the program. In return for their perseverance they met people, learned social skills they had lacked and, for the first time, started to feel like a part of something. In Carlos' words,

> I stuck with it because there were a lot of new people I was not so alone. Old teenagers--Henry and Jose--were gone, and I knew Richard. He was the only person I really felt comfortable with. Everybody was nervous 'cause there were new people. In the summer I became a worker. I felt like an old-timer. The program became part of me because I grew up with it and it helped me. And then I said, "If it helped me a little then maybe I can do the same for the kids that are in the same position that I was." So I said, "Okay, I'll stick with it and I'll help the kids in Unitas." I guess that's what made me so much a part of Unitas. Doc became a big part of my life, made a big difference. At home, nothing was stable for me.

Richard reiterates Carlos' feelings of alienation before he became involved in Unitas. He speaks of how, on Fox Street, where he lived at the time,

> ...everybody was involved in their own thing. There were different little groups. Doc brought the groups together. The block was brought together. We were all there together for the purpose of seeing Doc and the art therapist and Ted, one of the teen workers. We all joked around together and talked.

Richard and Carlos were the first of the current inner-circle workers to have entered Unitas. Each describes the attraction of Unitas in personal and emotional terms, pointing to the important role Eismann played in drawing him into the program. Both also name Henry and Jose, earlier inner-circle teens, though in different ways. Carlos speaks of how, by the time he became involved as a teenager, Henry and Jose were no longer in the program, thereby lessening his anxiety about being a newcomer. Richard, on the other hand, names Henry and Jose, along with Eismann, as the people who had been most important to him in his early days in Unitas. Though neither Carlos nor Richard was brought into Unitas by these older teens, they were clearly influential. This trend of older workers affecting younger teens continues.

Perhaps the best place to observe the influence of the more experienced workers is in the area of recruitment and support of new teen workers. Carlos was directly responsible for bringing three other teenagers, who eventually became inner-circle workers, into Unitas. But not all introductions lead to the kinds of commitment that the inner-circle workers express about Unitas. The personal network provided the route for teenagers into Unitas but it was not sufficient to keep them there. Once acquainted with the program, these workers unanimously describe the personal need the program filled.

George has been in Unitas since 1974, when he was sixteen. In 1979 he went to college, with plans to study psychology. When asked to describe his first experiences with Unitas, George responds:

> I was invited by Carlos and his brothers (two of Carlos' brothers were involved in Unitas for a time but dropped out) but what really attracted me was the new experience. It was something new, in terms of meeting with a group of teenagers my age, a little older, just to experience sitting together and just talking and relating to each other without getting into fights or arguments even though people disagree with each other. There was an openness. There was a chance for everyone to say what they felt like saying. It was a shocking experience, it was something that was very new...in terms of just being yourself. Natural. Not having to put up a front or an image. The sharing of a closeness with the people who are there.

Juan, too, speaks of how he felt he could get something he needed "because of the different aspects of my personality at that time." Juan describes himself as "shy and not too sure of myself"--a description that his inner-circle friends often give of themselves. Before he went to Unitas, Juan spoke at length with Carlos' brother about what the program would offer him:

> One of the things that he said was that if you came and you became a parent, or just a member, the entire group would help you get over any problems or any hangups you have. And anytime you needed any help or something, there would always be someone there to help you. There was something there that I needed and I knew that if I stuck around long enough I was gonna get that.

Two prominent themes run through the self-portraits of inner-circle members. First, they tended to be shy and somewhat alienated teenagers when they heard about Unitas from one or more friends already involved in and committed to the program. Second, by the time each worker had decided to participate in Unitas seriously, he had determined that he had a personal need that the program could fulfill. Usually he articulates this as a need for friendship with other people who will listen caringly to his feelings and offer help with his problems.

We asked the teenagers to compare the way they were when they first came to Unitas to the way they are now. The contrasts between the inner-circle workers' answers and the marginal teenagers' answers point to subtle lessons learned by more experienced and committed workers, and not yet by others. George's serious humor epitomizes the sentiments of all the inner-circle workers. In a high-pitched soft voice he says "shy and weak" to characterize his pre-Unitas self. He follows this with a deep resounding half-sung "macho man." Richard, hearing George's characterization, adds, "That speaks for all of us."

George expounds on his first brief description:

> That was it for us coming into a place very shy, scared, being not even aware of anyone else, and being very touchy. As you notice, now I'm outgoing, speak up, aggressive and very charming! I can get my point across. If I see something that I want I can now strive for it. It was an asset in helping me relate to people and gave me a clearer understanding of myself and other people which made it a lot easier. I use mostly the skills of just listening and empathizing and trying to relate to people and I understand where they're coming from or how they feel and whatever it is that I want in terms of making a relationship, in terms of talking, touching. It's simpler now, easier for me to do this.

Richard, an acknowledged leader of Unitas, has on numerous occasions, led the Thursday extended family circle meetings and the symbolic parents meeting which immediately follows. During the summer of 1979 he held the position of Crew Chief of most of the teenagers assigned to Unitas. In 1980 he was selected by Eismann and Stekas, with other inner-circle workers, to become trainers of other teens and Unitas workers. It is all the more surprising, therefore, to hear Richard describe his past self in the following way:

> I was shy, not certain about things, not a leader but a follower, dependent. Now, I'm a little overexagger-

> ated, a little overbearing, too aggressive sometimes. I can see myself as a leader if need be. I hate being a follower. I'm more dependent on myself. Let me deal with things myself. Even in my growth in Unitas I was dependent on Doc, Henry and Jose. There was always someone there.

The enjoyment that Richard clearly gets from being independent and a leader allows us to speculate about the fact that none of the people he has brought into Unitas have become inner-circle workers. As potential usurpers of his power, they perhaps threaten his position of leadership.

Other teenagers, not in the influential core group, respond similarly when asked to describe personal changes that they have experienced since entering Unitas. Most of the teenagers point to how they have learned to get along better with other people since joining Unitas. Tom, now 15 and in Unitas for two years, describes changes he perceives in himself:

> I used to be very shy. I didn't like to talk to anybody. The way I used to deal with a problem -- I wouldn't talk about it. I'm not shy any more. Sometimes I might be shy, but not as much as I used to be. It helped me out of it. I can cope with people better. I never could cope with people older than me or younger than me. I couldn't stand kids younger than me, but now that's everything, every little kid next to me.

Gaining self-confidence is expressed by many of the teenagers, whatever their status in the program, as a positive aspect of being in Unitas, whether in relations with their peers, older teenagers or young children.

Unitas has also helped teenagers to adjust to American life, a function never explicitly addressed either by Eismann or by the inner-circle workers. Peter, initially attracted by the sports and girls, describes what it was like for him coming to New York with his parents and siblings from Puerto Rico when he was six years old and the changes he has since experienced:

> I came from Puerto Rico in 1970. I was kind of young and got used to the Bronx the way it was. The first day I came to school, I had a fight. At that time it was the Puerto Ricans against the blacks and the whites. That's the way it felt at that time. When I came over here and I started getting older, at first this guy that was black said, "Do you wanna come?" I said, "Oh, sh--." He was telling me this! Other

> blacks asked me at the time and I started getting used to them and then I got along with them. Black, white, brown, whatever color, I don't care if they were purple! Not all blacks were enemies, but mostly all. When I first came here I went into school and this kid banged me over the head with a ruler and then started laughing. And I started talking Spanish. The dude would be snapping and I didn't know what he was saying. Then this other kid that was Puerto Rican translated to Spanish. I picked up a book and slapped him over the head and we started fighting.... Before I didn't use thought so much. I think about it now, I go to somebody else and think things out and talk things out. If it still don't work, I try talking to him again. I usually try it three times. If that don't work, I go back to the old way.

Although the lessons of Unitas -- of talking things out to resolve problems and having self-confidence to speak your mind -- have been well-learned, most teenages (not inner-circle workers) agree with Peter that if you can't get your point across, the final, preferred solution is fighting. Talking with an adversary or a friend is one way to win an argument but fighting is still viewed as a legitimate approach to follow. In this regard, inner-circle workers do not speak of fighting as a legitimate resolution of conflict, although all of them have been involved in physical fights.

The friendship networks that the teenagers maintain are particularly important in understanding both the degree of commitment of the workers and the maintenance of their ties to Unitas and, through Unitas, to one another. Inner-circle workers name one another as their closest friends. More marginal teenagers claim that their friends come primarily from school, play and the street. Inner-circle workers spend much of their non-Unitas time visiting with other inner-circle workers. Other teenagers do not. This fact may help account for difficulties the less experienced, less involved teens may have in resolving conflicts with their friends and acquaintances, that is, people, we may assume, who have not had the benefit of Unitas training in personal relations.

Eismann has encouraged closeness among the inner-circle workers by inviting them to his country house. The purpose of this house, according to Eismann, is to reward teenagers who have been doing a particularly admirable job in Unitas. This usually includes the inner-circle workers, with the exception of Terry, the only female in this group, who has never been to visit. Other teenagers who we have classified as up-and-coming in the hierarchy, have also received invitations to the house for a weekend, which they eagerly accept. The visits, from the description of these workers, sometimes take on the atmosphere of summit talks. Several of these core workers proudly say that they often act as advisers to Eismann, keeping him informed of the needs of Unitas teenage workers and children.

The male orientation of Unitas is again apparent in these visits to Eismann's lake house. Although Stekas could theoretically accompany a group of teenage girls on a special trip, she does not share Eismann's "after hours" commitment to the Unitas program or workers. The teenage girls are well aware of how they have been slighted in the past and it is this dissatisfaction that led to the formation of a female therapy and support group.

In 1979, a number of the more experienced youth began college studies and faced a host of personal problems unknown to them previously. One by one, they began to turn to Lynn Stekas to talk about their concerns until she decided to bring these teenagers together to discuss their shared problems. A college support group emerged, made up of half a dozen young men either in college or about to enter. They decided to restrict participation in their weekly group to males, with the group to be led by Stekas. Meanwhile, the young women of Unitas -- the teenage girls in college or with college aspirations -- decided, also encouraged by Stekas, to form a group of their own, which also would meet once a week with Stekas. Until that time, these teenage girls had met only informally, as friends, without a structured place within Unitas equivalent to the male support group.

In summation, a number of factors serve to distinguish more involved, influential workers in Unitas from less committed, less powerful teenagers. Inner-circle workers are not necessarily older than other workers, nor have they necessarily spent more time in Unitas. They do, however, invest more of their time in Unitas, attending and running meetings, supervising other teens and simply maintaining their own friendships. These friendships tend to involve other inner-circle workers, thus reinforcing the exclusivity of this group.

Related to this, inner-circle teens, the backbone of the Unitas structure, are firmly committed to and have incorporated well the Unitas credo in ways that the less committed teenagers have not. In doing this, they have also learned therapeutic skills in handling children and dealing with interpersonal problems. Such expertise may well account for the popularity they enjoy among the children, who are more attracted to their symbolic family groupings than to those of less experienced teenagers.

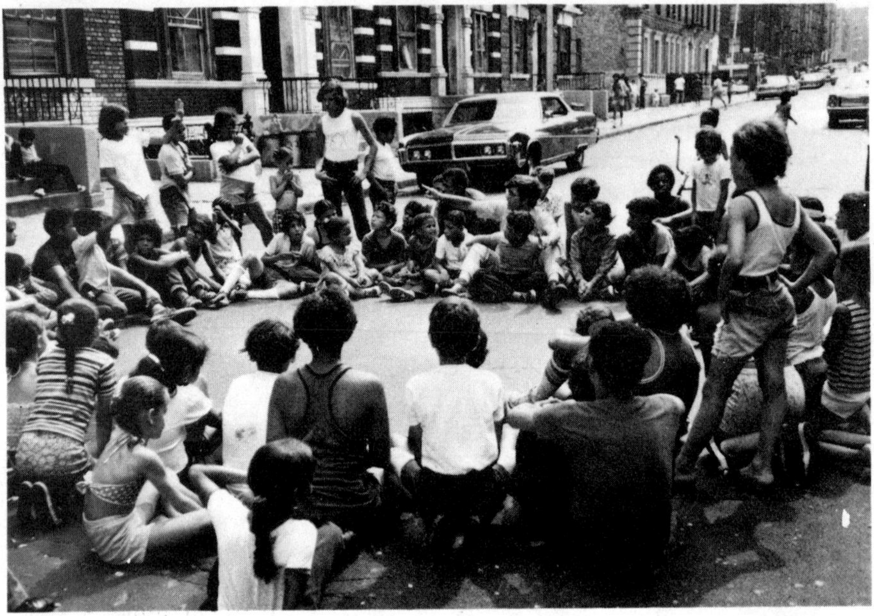

PLATE 7. The "family circle" as therapeutic community: "People are merely people, with the feelings of any one human being echoed in some way in every other human being."

VI

CONCLUSIONS

The theoretical and organizational underpinnings of the Unitas Therapeutic Community provide a basis for the discussion of two key issues: the "success" of Unitas as a mental health program and the feasibility and desirability of replicating such a program.

If success is measured in terms of desired psychological change in the children as the result of participation in Unitas, then at present we lack the data necessary to arrive at a conclusion. The question of improvement in the mental health status of the children can only be answered by the results of carefully designed, experimentally oriented psychometric studies. This was not our purpose in conducting the present investigation of Unitas. Our purpose was to explore and clarify systematically the institutional structure, value system and social processes imbedded in Unitas. Therefore, what we propose regarding psychological change among the children must remain on the level of a hypothesis. We shall argue presently that the children in Unitas are likely to change psychologically in the direction postulated by the program.

We must insist, however, that the success of a program such as Unitas is not exclusively a matter of bringing about psychological change in the children. Such change is but one measure of success. Thus, if success is measured by the consistency of purpose and the congruence between the theoretical model and the social structure, then, Unitas is, indeed, successful. This monograph is replete with data demonstrating the close relationship between the theoretical or ideal model(s) of a therapeutic community which guided the creation of Unitas as a tangible social organization. The structures which it creates are planned, instilling social processes that are also planned.

As a structure, Unitas provides its participants with safe and carefully organized after-school and summer activities. The value of this function should not be taken lightly when we consider that Unitas does its work in the South Bronx, an area which has come to symbolize urban decay in the United States. It is an area lacking in parks, playgrounds, planned recreational and educational programs for children. Unitas' combination of psychotherapeutic and recreational activities offers children a set of participatory experiences as an alternative to the street.

The alternative it offers children is also relevant to an evaluation of the organization's success. To join Unitas means to be integrated into a purposefully constructed network of social relations enmeshing the children, the teenagers serving as symbolic parents and therapists, the program's director and the administrator, and the other participants. The network has been pieced together by design to bond each person to another person in the interest of intimate and nurturent relations. In turn, the interactions of persons in the network are guided by the therapeutic goal of mutual help, a goal which has been instilled and is repeatedly reinforced through the incessant teachings of the program's creator and director, and is perpetuated and given face-to-face meaning by the therapeutically trained teenagers serving as symbolic parents.

A point should be emphasized which our data repeatedly confirm: the symbolic parents maintain contact with the children away from Unitas, and retain the forms of the therapeutic and parenting interactions with the children that they have learned at Unitas. This process is facilitated -- indeed, it is made possible -- by the fact that the symbolic parents and children live near each other in the same neighborhoods. Thus, the network of social relations created at the very core of Unitas' official activities functions away from Unitas in the nearby neighborhoods of the South Bronx, at whatever time of the day or night the children and symbolic parents meet. The client in need of help does not separate himself or herself from the source of help located inside the four walls of a clinic. A product of Unitas' efforts is that help-giving extends to the periphery of the network in the familiar settings of the children's neighborhoods.

Geographically larger than the site of the official Unitas and active at all hours, the network exposes the participants to a coherently planned set of opportunities for socialization. At the heart of the socialization experience are a set of cultural values symbolically expressed through the repeated rituals of meetings, such as the breaking of the bread and the feeding of the children. The values focus upon desired behavior. At Unitas it is good to share and to help others in time of need; it is good to be disciplined; it is good to be polite; it is good to be self-controlled and not resort to physical violence; it is good to be responsible; and so on through an array of desired behavior. Obviously, Unitas does not create such values. Rather, it selects them from the broader cultural context, giving particular emphasis to those values pertaining to the form, content, and nuances of interpersonal relations; therefore, they are values likely to have psychotherapeutic meaning. Through repetition the values come to be associated with the symbol of human unity which is Unitas. The associations formed, the values are then linked to therapeutically relevant skills and procedures which trace to the writings of Alfred Adler and Maxwell Jones and to modern concepts of family therapy. If Unitas can make one claim to uniqueness it is that all of this is imbedded in an outreach psychotherapeutic program whose core organizing principle is the symbolic nuclear and extended family. Ironically, the fiction of such symbolic families is what gives reality to the values and skills forming part of the socialization process.

Two additional observations should be made. The first related to therapy. Without placing explicit intellectual or ideological emphasis upon issues of cultural and ethnic identity, Unitas employs workers who are from similar backgrounds and who share the same stoops, gutters, schools, and friends. Children perceive role models from their own community. The teenagers and workers speak Spanish with children and families, translating the concepts and techniques they have been taught into the idiom of the people. It is important to note in this regard, however that sharing the same culture and language does not of itself insure a successful community outreach effort. Eismann was unsuccessful in his earlier work at a Bronx community mental health center with community paraprofessionals. More recently, on four separate occasions in four years, Unitas attempted to form mothers' groups to discuss issues brought up by the mothers themselves. Despite the fact that Spanish-speaking paraprofessionals were used to recruit the mothers and babysitting services were offered, no more than two or three mothers in an entire school expressed an interest in these groups. Commonality of culture and language is no substitute for the difficult task of daily work at the grassroots level of urban life in the interest of developing stable networks to serve the predispositions and needs of the participants.

The second observation is that Unitas combines treatment and prevention in addressing the needs of disturbed and normal children by stressing the values of human interdependence and reciprocity. In order to teach help-giving skills, teenagers are given help. The training of the teenagers is itself treatment, tapping into personal and family experience for the purpose of better understanding the children. Confidence is gained from mastery of new skills and knowledge. The outlook upon family life which is developed becomes part of a process of anticipatory socialization into future roles as parents. The outlook is optimistically based upon the value of human beings caring for each other and of how misunderstandings can be resolved through open, verbal communication rather than through physical violence. Eventually, the "patients" become "therapists." Unitas does not foster the continuing dependence of the children upon the teenagers or the teenagers upon the program's director. As the life-cycle changes and the socialization process continues, natural leaders emerge from the teenage group, form the core group, and begin to take on autonomous leadership functions.

Thus, the construction of a far-reaching neighborhood network, patterned according to concepts of symbolic families, provides a vehicle for socialization experiences relevant to values and therapeutic skills. And, even though the children and teenagers drawn into Unitas are probably those likely to be congenial to the program, we believe the desired psychological change in children does occur. Why? To be a part of the Unitas network is to be governed by a highly active system of sanctions which rewards the valued behavior and the mastery of skills while discouraging undesirable conduct. External pressures of this kind are likely to make the withdrawn child more sociable, the acting-out child more serene, and likely, too, to instill control and restraint into children given to bizarre behavior. The hypothesis that the desired psychological change occurs is more than just plausible because it is based upon an essentially credible theory of the type of social system likely to influence psychological functioning. We are not in the realm of hypothesis, however, in pointing to the fact that Unitas as a social system tangibly replicates prevailing views of an effective therapeutic community, offers children an alternative to the streets of the South Bronx, integrates the children into a wide-ranging supportive network, and offers them socialization opportunities for the development of functional skills and values.

In discussing the problem of replicability, we are faced with two questions. First, are attempts at replicating Unitas worthwhile? And, second, is it possible to replicate Unitas? The answer to the first question already has been foreshadowed throughout this manuscript in what has been an essentially favorable account of the program. Yes, attempts at replicating Unitas are worthwhile. The answer is based upon the authors' values which coincide with the objectives of the program, and upon the program's success according to the terms of discussion just presented. While we believe stronger efforts should be made to incorporate the participation and leadership of girls and women into the program, and at the same time recently have felt a nudging discomfort that Unitas may be diluting its primary group character in the interest of bureaucratic procedures, the program as a whole merits applause.

Its worthiness is accentuated by the context in which it functions, the South Bronx, an area which is so barren of the organizational life and amenities customary to the lives of middle-class children.

The consideration of the second question, the replicability of Unitas, must begin with the cost of the program. The program has always had to function within a strictly limited budget. From June 1, 1979 to May 30, 1980, 413 people participated in the program. This figure includes children, parents, and workers participating in one or more of the following: the tutoring program, art groups, individual therapy, the Unitas circle, therapeutic play groups, group therapy for teenagers, family therapy and family work. The total budget for that year was $88,900, yielding a per capita treatment cost of $215. If, to the total budget, we add contributions in goods and services of $47,782,[17] the per capita figure climbs to $331.

Unfortunately, we lack comparable data for programs similar to Unitas. However, if we turn to the costs of a program aimed, as is Unitas, toward the maintenance of children within their biological families, in their own communities, we find that Unitas' costs are, using the most conservative figures, one-fourth of those normally expected. Thus, in 1976, the Child Welfare League of America determined that the cost of providing a preventive service for one child for one year was approximately $1,200, as compared to the nearly $6,600 annual costs of maintaining a child in foster care.[18]

Unlike other mental health agencies, Unitas has not directed its limited funds toward the hiring of highly trained mental health personnel. From its inception, Unitas has been a grassroots movement based upon the social mobilization and training of teenagers to serve as therapists and symbolic parents. It did not emerge as a bureaucratic response to a set of federal prescriptions or funding opportunities relevant to mental health. On the contrary,

[17] In 1979-1980, these included contributions from St. Athanasius of space ($6,000 per year), the Youth Employment Program which supported 12 Unitas workers (18,900 per year), the Urban Corps which supported 12 workers ($10,300 per year), the National Institute of Mental Health which provided stipends to three MSW students ($9,000 each year), and teenagers who volunteered 1194 hours of their time to work at Unitas (at $3 per hour = $3,582).

[18] Jones, Mary Ann *et al.*, 1976, *A Second Chance for Families*, Research Center, Child Welfare League of America, Inc. Such comparisons should, ideally, consider factors which would bear directly on a careful determination of costs and their comparability, including overhead, length and type of treatment offered, the makeup of the patient population, and personnel costs. For example, we cannot provide a per family cost for Unitas since family therapy is only one component of the larger treatment program not budgetarily separable from other therapy components. Most preventive programs directed towards children view the biological family and not the children as cases, whereas Unitas considers children as cases. Thus, not only must we examine overall operating costs of the program but the ways in which these costs are determined and allocated.

Eismann had to disconnect himself from the community mental health center where he worked and turn to the streets of the South Bronx to piece together step-by-uncertain-step the social relations among teenagers which would eventually culminate in Unitas. He capitalized upon the human resources of the South Bronx by forming friendships, nurturing and training the teenagers who came to Unitas, some first as children, others as teenagers. Curiously, it is Unitas' innovative use of already existing human resources at the neighborhood grassroot level which enables it to operate on such a low budget. The innovative use of such resources, therefore, accounts for its low budget and at the same time *defines* the essential character of Unitas as a therapeutic organization. Both are inextricably intertwined.

Unitas' comparatively low budget ought not to invite the conclusion that it is easily replicable. To the contrary, Unitas attains a low budget as a result of a complicated primary group process at the neighborhood grassroot level aimed at socially mobilizing teenagers into the joint roles of therapist and symbolic parent. The issue of replicability *must* be seen in relation to such a process. Before we continue to examine this point, however, two observations are in order. First, we must stress that Unitas cannot be reduced to a "how to do it" manual, complete with step-by-step instructions for easy replication. This observation is in need of emphasis because of the current penchant for simplistic, programmatic recipes or prescriptions addressing complex mental health needs. Secondly, the feasibility of replicating the Unitas program, wholly or in part, presents a difficult problem which must be considered as logically separate from that of the value of attempting such a replication. In fact, no easy answer can be given to the issue of replication because the question presupposes more than we now know about the circumstances surrounding future efforts at replication. We cannot discount Unitas' particular history within a specific social and cultural context, directed and managed by particular personnel. But we would need to consider, too, the goals of replication, the context in which replication would take place, the personnel who would develop and run the program, the clientele they would serve and other structural variables which might affect program establishment and success. Such factors would need to be carefully examined before replication could be accomplished.

We shall proceed on the assumption, however, that it is instructive to speculate upon the degree to which the Unitas organizational structure can be reproduced, provided that specific amenable circumstances are present. Our speculations will be based upon the concept of bureaucracy. If a program or organization is highly bureaucratized, by definition, it will contain an explicit hierarchical structure complete with the rights and obligations of a circumscribed set of status roles. Max Weber describes the purest type of bureaucratic structure as functioning under one "supreme chief of the organization" whose "authority pertains to a sphere of legal 'competence'."[19] The management of a bureaucracy is based on written documents which set forth the fixed, official jurisdictional areas and the administrative rules by which they are regulated.[20] The bureaucratic administrative staff member is appointed and functions according to criteria which stress the technical qualifications necessary to perform satisfactorily within a position or a "sphere of competence" clearly defined and hierarchically contextualized. The office he holds, viewed as his principal occupation and considered a career, determines appropriate behavior which is strictly controlled. The individual is contractually employed and paid a fixed salary graded according to rank in the hierarchy. In addition, the individual has no ownership in the means of administration. Within the organization he is replaceable, judged primarily in terms of his competency to function in accordance with the duties of his position.

The highly explicit, prescriptive, rule-governed nature of bureaucracy renders it amenable to replication. It would seem, then, that the more highly bureaucratized the structure of an organization, the more easily it can be reproduced. Unitas, however, is an emergent, grassroot organization and, as such, it falls substantially short of the criteria established by Weber for an ideal bureaucracy. Although there is an internally consistent philosophy underlying the program, it is unwritten, as are the rules governing the behaviors of the members of the organization. Management in this case is based on the application of a set of general principles of human behavior -- minimally distinguishable from the substantive teachings of the program -- within a loosely organized structure.

The appointment of staff within Unitas is only partially on the basis of prescribed technical qualifications. The teenagers and social work students must demonstrate sensitivity to the children with whom they work, and a willingness to become committed to the work of the program, i.e., to the goals of creating bonds of friendship with staff, teenagers, and especially, with children. This is not a simple task, nor is it one for which a person can readily receive technical training beforehand. There are many teenagers and staff members who have not been successful in Unitas, either

[19] Weber, Max. *The Theory of Social and Economic Organization*. New York: Free Press, 1947, pp. 333-334.

[20] Gerth, H.H. and C.Wright Mills. *From Max Weber: Essays in Sociology*. New York: Oxford University Press, 1958, pp. 196-198.

because of their own discomfort within the program or because they were perceived as misfits or deadbeats.

Within the structure of the Unitas extended family circle the duties of the Unitas teenager and staff member are more clearly established. As surrogate mothers, fathers, aunts and uncles, participants have an understanding of their responsibilities. In practically all cases, however, the position which is held is not viewed as the major occupation of the individual, or his or her career. Unitas' desire to have unpaid staff attend regularly does not alter the fact that they can exert little influence, outside of peer pressure, over these volunteers. Paid staff are in the minority. Salaries are not offered to all workers within a given rank, nor are salaries within a rank necessarily the same for all paid workers. Paid staff are usually teenagers who, after many years of dedicated volunteering at Unitas, receive part-time compensation for their efforts. As indicated above, however, without exception, these teenagers continue to volunteer time to Unitas work.

An important criterion for bureaucratic administrative staff is the ability to substitute one qualified staff member for another equally qualified, according to established criteria. The duties involved in managing various aspects of Unitas are not clearly and irrevocably delegated either to the director or to the administrator. Each takes on those activities and responsibilities which he or she is best able to do. Were a key individual in this organization to leave, his or her replacement would undoubtedly cause a change in the program. Although the social work students are replaced each year, as are various consultants and specialists who work for Unitas on a part-time basis, the core of teenagers who devote their time to the program cannot be so easily replaced. Friendship with peers and with neighborhood children can be neither bureaucratically created, ordered nor maintained.

In sum, Unitas does not fulfill selected bureaucratic criteria relevant to the possibility of its replication: it is loosely prescriptive of status-relevant behaviors in the context of unwritten norms; the recruitment of persons deemphasizes technical qualifications in favor of attributes associated with friendship and sociability; the core group of teenagers are neither fully salaried nor is their position as surrogate parents viewed as a major career; and, perhaps most important, the bonds of friendship enmeshing the children and teenagers into the network are crescive and achieved through primary group processes, not bureaucratically enacted as a result of externally imposed prescriptions. This means, therefore, that one teenager cannot replace another teenager because each teenager/symbolic parent is part of a broader network which enmeshes him or her in a uniquely earned, neighborhood based configuration of friendship with the symbolic children. If there is one element distinguishing the Unitas structure, it is precisely this configuration of friendship patterns. They are the planned by-products of socially mobilizing teenagers as human resources in the South Bronx.

Unitas, of course, displays some elements of bureaucracy. Since its inception, Eismann has been dependent upon outside funding to maintain the program, even minimally. And indeed, it was the pressures of economic survival which pushed Unitas to hire an administrator, a bookkeeper, and a secretary -- personnel important to the administering of an agency in ways conducive to the securing and maintenance of financial backing. With this increased bureaucratization has come a shift in Eismann's position within Unitas. Teenagers who were personally trained and closely supervised and supported by Eismann have begun to assume new roles, establishing program pieces by themselves, running meetings that previously had been run only by Eismann. They have also begun to turn for assistance not just to Eismann but to Stekas, a social worker with professional training and authority in Unitas. Regardless of the shift in Eismann's role and economic circumstances, there has been a built-in flexibility in areas of personnel and programming which has consistently characterized the program and its work. People are expected to pitch in when they are needed and to help others do the same, thus having the effect of dissipating alienation which may accompany an inflexible hierarchically organized program.

Whether this evolution is necessary for the success of Unitas or a program like it is one factor which bears on the question of replicability. Where then are we left with respect to the question of replicability? Even though Unitas lacks those aspects of bureaucracy which lend themselves to replication, we have determined that it would be impossible to transplant features or components of Unitas to other contexts, separate from the historical richness of the original program. This already has been accomplished within Unitas and outside of Unitas. Within Unitas, in 1980, an afterschool program was developed and implemented by teenage workers in the local public elementary school. This program, based on the Unitas concept and using Unitas techniques, assembles teenagers, now participating in Unitas, one evening each week. Outside of Unitas, educators and mental health workers, trained by Eismann in Unitas methods, have successfully applied the "circle" concept in their work with children. Thus, the analytical distinction made between the historical events leading to the creation of Unitas and the structure that was formed can be made to have operational meaning.

To fit one component of Unitas to a specific need in evidence in a nearby locale, and to do this by drawing upon the experienced persons in the program, presents no serious difficulty. However, it is quite another matter to attempt the replication of the program in its entirety or substantially in the scope of its function, in a setting distant from or different from the present context of its functions. Even if we make an assumption we believe to be correct, that the values emphasized by Unitas transcend local cultural boundaries, thus lending themselves to different subcultural variants -- and the children's needs in the neighborhood settings designated for replication are comparable to those of the South Bronx children -- the task of such replication would indeed be formidable, although probably not impossible to perform. Assuming a supportive and congenial institutional environment, the essential task -- the *sine qua non* of the effort -- would be, once again, the social mobilization of neighborhood teenagers into a motivated and therapeutically trained *cadre* of symbolic parents abidingly interested in the welfare of children in their neighborhoods, and profoundly convinced of the worthiness of the Unitas undertaking. It is difficult to conceive of how this could be done, without doing what Eismann did at the very beginning: forming friendships with the teenagers in the streets, alleys, vacant lots, and stairways of the South Bronx, and learning how to use the indigenous social organization of this territory.

We are left with one final observation. Direct participation in the program beforehand is probably necessary, if the goal is to replicate the program in a substantive part or in its entirety. Direct participation yields knowledge by acquaintance which is not entirely reducible to explicitly rendered sets of prescriptions on how to accomplish therapeutic goals. Direct participation provides a clinical sense of the expressive components of the healing process, and the clear recognition of the need for the commitment to an ethic of helping other persons, whether that ethic be rooted in religious, humanistic or psychotherapeutic beliefs.